PLAY PIERCING

PLAY PIERCING

BY DEBORAH ADDINGTON

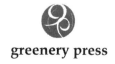

greenery press

CONTENTS

Welcome 1

Section 1: Preparation 5
    Introduction..*5*
    What is Play Piercing?......................................*8*
    Play Piercing Isn't for Everyone..................*12*
    Risk..*12*
    Negotiation...*16*
    FAQ...*18*

Section 2: Anatomy 27
    Anatomy of Needles.......................................*27*
    Sizes and Gauges..*29*
    Anatomy of Skin...*30*
    Piercing Sites...*33*

Section 3: Perforation 37
    Cleaning Surfaces..*38*
    Cleaning Skin...*39*
    Set Your Tray...*39*
    Procedure...*41*
    Insertion..*41*
    How Deep?..*46*
    How Long a Pass?...*47*

Subdermal Sensation Techniques *47*

Decorating *49*

Section 4: Tidying Up   55

Removal *55*

Clean Up After Yourself *57*

Aftercare *59*

Troubleshooting *61*

Basic Wound Care *63*

Section 5: Advanced Practices   67

Play Piercing and Blood Play *67*

Nipples and Genitals *76*

Nipples *77*

Male Genitals *79*

Female Genitals *80*

Appendix A: Universal Precautions   85

Appendix B: Resources   89

Supplies *90*

Appendix C: A Complete Play Piercing Kit   93

Acknowledgments   97

About the Author   99

WELCOME

Welcome to *Play Piercing!* I'm terribly pleased you have chosen to expand your awareness and knowledge of this happy subject. I salute your adventuring spirit. Before we get to the juicy bits, let's get some business out of the way.

This is a guide for the novice play piercer and is no substitute for hands-on education and training. This is intended to serve as a beginner's map to the joys of play piercing and should be valued accordingly. This is not a guide to exotic piercings, temporary or permanent. Instruction by a qualified and competent play or body piercer is recommended for all advanced activities. Please, do not ever use anything other than a sterile needle for play piercing and follow the Universal Precautions listed in the back of this book to reduce the chances of infection and cross-contamination. The life and limb you save may be your own.

I wish also to inform you that in addition to the physical risks of play piercing, there's a mental challenge embedded in this text. Throughout this book, I use some loaded words. I'm going to talk about things like a skinsuit, spirit, soul, the Universe, the Divine, the All (some people call it God). I'm going to talk about loaded subjects, things like personal responsibility and communication. The challenge is for you to unload those words and subjects, to take judgments and opinions out of your response and to truly look at the information provided herein. It's fine with me if you don't like the wrapping paper this information comes in, but do yourself a favor and don't throw the gift out with the giftwrap.

I love play piercing. It's one of my favorite intensities, and I love it equally (though differently) on both ends of a needle. I love being the piercer, the one penetrating and crafting. I don't consider myself a masochist, but I do love being a pincushion, the receptive, doted upon, perforated person who gets to sit back and enjoy. I love blood: the sight, smell and taste of it. With play piercing, I get intensity *and* blood: an excellent package deal. I wrote this book in hopes of helping people to share my passion and do so with as little risk as possible. In order to share my passion I must also share fact and belief; we begin this adventure with some belief.

We are composite beings. There's a thinking, intellectual brainy part we call the mind. There's a feeling, intuitive, animating spark that we usually name spirit or soul. And then there's the vehicle, the container that all the parts fit in: I call that a skinsuit. It's a shield, an environmental interface, a mobility device and many other fine things. I perceive my skinsuit as a cross between a holy temple and a kickass amusement park.

Because your skinsuit does so much, it's easy to make the mistake of thinking that you *are* your skinsuit. You're not. You're inextricably connected to your skinsuit, but you don't stop there. You are the being that lives inside your skinsuit, and when you do something to your insides it affects your skinsuit. For example, too much stress can give you a heart attack, or cause an ulcer. Your mind and spirit are the primary experiencers of stress, but it's your skinsuit that most reflects the relationship of the individual to stressors. Likewise, when you do something to your skinsuit, it affects your mind and spirit. During an intense energy exchange, the mundane world falls away, taking you on adventures in your innerscape, places your skinsuit alone can't take you. Play piercing is a swell example of something you can do to and with your skinsuit that can result in deep and profound alterations to your insides.

This book has two purposes: its primary function is as an instructional guide to the act of play piercing, teaching how to correctly and accurately put needles in a skinsuit. That's technical information and there's plenty of it.

This book's second but no less significant purpose is to open the door to making play piercing a part of your own spiritual, kinky practice. Kink is the one of the most gorgeous ways we have of mixing skinsuit, mind and soul; it is my privilege to offer you, through this text, the distillation of my own experience.

The individual seeks reunion with the All. We want to touch God and be touched by God, the All That Is, the Source from which we all come. Sex and kink are a perfect mirror for that pursuit. When we get out of our way, we are connected to the All. When we play with others, we give ourselves the opportunity to experience unity with another skinsuit; that union mirrors the union to the All. Skinsuits need other skinsuits to create the connection, the body between them. Just as the individual seeks reunion with the divine, the Everything, the All, so do skinsuits seek union with one another. Play piercing provides a focus and impetus for connection, integration and expansion.

Play piercing is a versatile tool for pain and pleasure, skin sensation and soul sensation. As with any experience or symbol set, your mileage with play piercing may vary. As both examples and illustrations, you'll find vignettes in *italics* throughout the text. Each vignette is a little piece of real experience; none of the stories are fiction. May you enjoy them as much as the participants did; may you use them as seeds for the crop of your own experiences. I invite you to offer a thought of thanks to those who've shared with you.

Some of you will assume that the information in this basic reference will be enough for you to deduce how to perform the more intricate, complicated and advanced piercings. That is not the case. Genitals aren't the same as, say, biceps, and they will differ per gender and per individual. The face is a world unto itself, with the ways it's rigged for blood and nerves. Considering suspension piercings? The information here is not near enough to what you need to know to be involved in large hooks or suspension. For all of the advanced techniques, you need more than basic anatomy and the basic techniques in this book. I understand that some of you are going to do whatever you're going to do but please, *please* do not do it because you *think* you know something. Get educated. Learn all you can about human anatomy (which will also make you a better all-around lover). Make clear, conscious and informed choices about play piercing and how you weave it into your own sexual or spiritual practice. There's abundant magic and alchemy in play piercing; you get to add that on your own.

And now, on to the juicy bits.

Section 1: Preparation

Introduction

The first time anything sharp went through my skin, I was six. I stapled my finger to see what it felt like. It hurt like a sonofabitch, but I was intrigued by the pain, the frenzy of panic I felt about the injury and the blood.

The older I became, the more I learned about my skinsuit's mechanics. The more I learned, the more interested I became in discovering exactly what my skinsuit could do and how I could make it do more and more and more.

I was eleven the first time I put a needle in my skin. It was a sewing needle that I'd sharpened on an emery board and then heated with a match. I've never been much of a masochist; I figured the sharper the needle was, the less it would hurt. I'd seen my mother do the match thing, to sterilize a needle before remove splinters from my tender little fingers. This time, there was no splinter. There was nothing that needed to be removed from me, no foreign object requiring eviction. This time, I wanted to get at something. I wanted to experience a color that lurked just beneath my skin.

I knew from images and experience that people bled red. But at my wrists, just under my skin, were lines of blue. I'd read and heard the phrase "blue blood" used to refer to something of a higher class, a greater quality. I had an active fantasy life, and entertained the deliciously melodramatic notion that I had been kidnapped by the people who raised me, that I was perhaps estranged from a great legacy and its attendant mansion, servants, wealth. I considered that if I could prove myself to be one of those who bled blue, I'd be able to rejoin the ranks of my true and entitled people and escape the constraints of my 'family.' So I took that needle, sharp and clean as I knew how to get it, and stabbed towards the blue of possibility in my wrists.

I missed. Repeatedly.

I learned a lot about venipuncture from my mistakes. If you don't know what you're doing—and I sure as hell didn't--veins roll out from under you. I was frustrated that I couldn't get at the blue under my skin. Because I was a need-to-know type of child, I did some research. I was resolved to discover why there was blue under my skin, and how I could get at it. I found out that blue blood was blue because it had delivered its oxygen load and was removing toxins. I found out that even if I did manage to make that blue tube hold still long enough to tap it that it bled red, that all blood turns red as soon as it touches air. I bore a child's disappointment that my blood wasn't blue, but that disappointment ushered in a freedom to explore. I discovered that I had a profound connection to and affection for blood. I discovered that the container my blood came in could do some remarkable things and I wanted to learn how to master both blood and the container it came in.

Some years later, I was introduced to play piercing. I experienced the excitement of learning something new, and the relief of learning that there were others who shared my interest. I set about to learn all I could, studying anatomy, physiology and what little information there was (incomplete at best and dangerously incorrect at worst). I found teachers who could show me an increasingly intricate and delightful variety of techniques and playmates who let me practice on them. I've done scenes that involved a whole lot of needles and not much else, and I've had transcendent experiences involving only a few needles. I've done flesh pulls, and long to attempt a full-body horizontal suspension. As a vampire-style blood fetishist, I've used play piercing to feed my lust and taste for blood while simultaneously turning my donor into a work of art. Needles and a skinsuit are all the toys you need to play this game, but it may become much, much more than flesh and poke.

I'm not saying that play piercing *will* change your life. I'm saying it *can*. Play piercing may simply be the giving or receiving of needles and experiencing the physical sensations that result. Play piercing may be that element of ritual that connects you to others in a manner that reflects the individual's connection to the All. Whatever play piercing is for you, prepare for a journey of body, of mind, of taboo, of soul.

> I claimed the needle, made it a part of my hand. It felt right, an extension of my touch, my need to invade, my desire to penetrate. I felt for the right place, the asking of skin for the reception of metal. She shivered as I stabilized, tautened the skin. She felt the electricity spark between us as I lined the metal up with her body's lines. I corrected my angle, set the exit. With everything a breath away, I found her eyes, luminous and piercing. We were ready.
>
> "I'm going in on your third exhale from now. When that third breath leaves your body, my metal will take its place." I watched her step into herself, calculating, each breath a forever between now and needle.

The third breath went in; she held it, afraid of what would happen when it left, knowing she couldn't hold it forever. The third breath left and she was caught, impaled on the tip of my sharp love.

WHAT IS PLAY PIERCING?

On the surface, play piercing is the temporary subdermal insertion of sterile hypodermic needles for pleasure and pain (mostly the good kind, unless otherwise desired, of course). Most piercings done in play are surface-to-surface piercings, meaning that they go in and out of a flat or slightly curved surface, like an arm or the chest. Other piercings will go through a body part, such as an earlobe or a nipple. The technique for those parts is called pinch, because one pinches a section of tissue to pierce. Play piercing is a blood sport and should be treated with great care and respect, up to and including the observance of Universal Precautions, the medical standard for infectious risk reduction.

Play piercing is an activity appropriate to the deeper explorations of the connections between skin, psyche and soul. It is both vehicle and destination; it stands alone as a recreational activity or may be incorporated in ritual. It can focus your awareness down to the point of a needle or expand it to include the Universe, the All. It's one of those things that appears simple, even easy, on the outside but reveals startling complexity on closer examination. It beautifully, gracefully weaves into a BDSM context; it translates effortlessly into an act of sadism and just as easily becomes an act of submission. It can reflect one's dominance over another; it can be received as the fulfillment of masochism. It's a tool, an art, an undeniable source of immediate, demanding experience. Historically, it's been used as a rite of passage, punishment, a medical practice and a method of spiritual absolution. When needles are involved, everything else falls away. It's you, your other(s), and the needle. The stage for alchemy is set.

For some, the term "play piercing" has the ring of an oxymoron. How could having a needle slid beneath the skin be playful? How erotic or transcendent can it be to get punctured? Doesn't that *hurt*? And wait a minute — transcendent? How in the world could something like needles be part of a transcendent experience anyway?

For many of us, our only exposure to hypodermic needles is in a medical context and usually unpleasant. Getting a shot or having blood drawn are hardly erotic, sensuous experiences leading to an altered state of perception. For people traumatized by needles, this negative association can be difficult to break. Difficult, but not impossible; play piercing can dramatically change one's relationship to needles from something fearful and unpleasant to something delicious and sensuous

When we deny experience out of fear, we contract. We get smaller. It isn't the fear itself that makes us smaller; it's our reaction to the fear. When we surrender to sensations we're not sure we can manage, we get bigger in order to make room for them. Intensity forces us to expand and accommodate demanding, immediate sensations. Ever felt like your head or heart or other body part was about to explode during an intense energy exchange? That feeling of imminent explosion is your skinsuit shifting to make room for more of its invisible contents. I, and others like me, play with that phenomenon deliberately in the attempt to enlarge a capacity for pleasure and for the joyous act of expansion itself. It feels good to get bigger.

When we take the reins of control from another, we get bigger in order to hold and guide our travels with them. To achieve that level of mastery, a certain amount of self must be moved around in order to make room for the energies of another, a fascinating process in its own right. Play piercing, from either end of the needle, is a fabulous tool for opening places in the self, moving things around and making room for more.

Play piercing is socially taboo, physically challenging and psychologically edgy. We're not "supposed" to enjoy poking people with needles, or enjoy getting poked. Society seems to think that people who do that sort of thing are weird, danger-ous and possibly even sick. Taboos hold a great deal of power, and play piercing gives us access to that power, which we can then play with as we choose, using it for our own pleasure and evolution. Claiming one's power and using it in ways that make one happy is not sick; surrendering one's personal authority to inappropriate cultural, social or religious mandates is sick.

Chemically, play piercing triggers a deep-seated survival response abetted by a spike in brain chemical production. Your skinsuit perceives a threat, rushes itself with adrenaline and en-dorphins in preparation of a fight or a flight. If needed, extra resources for survival would be available. In the absence of a "real" threat, we get to sit back, relax and enjoy the rush.

There's also an edge of vulnerability in the mind when we do things that have inherent risk. The fears that arise when we face a risk give us the opportunity to transcend them, to become larger than our fears and bigger than we were before we overcame our fears. That altered perception, that transcendent state, is relatively easy to achieve with play piercing. It's not for everyone, but it's perfect for those in pursuit of transformation and transcendence.

If you're not into an holistic approach to pain, evolution and altered states of perception, you can always just play pierce for the sheer, joyful pain of it all, as well as the blood and the heat and the red and the sharp of it all. Sometimes a needle is just a needle and a pincushion is just a pincushion.

We indulge in play piercing to overcome, to be overwhelmed, to be washed away in a flood of our own chemistry and connection to another. We endure the poke and transmute the pain, empowered by transcending a challenging sensation and turning it into pleasure. We share an intimate, powerful exchange of energy by getting under someone's skin, or letting someone under ours. Partially because it's risky, play piercing is a rush. Its intensity doesn't feel quite like anything else. Play piercing is done for pain, for pleasure, for transcendent experience. It is done for bloodletting, for the opportunity to play with and consume that powerful, sacred elixir of life. It is done for decoration, from the patterning of needles to additions of dangly bits to lacing and "corsetry." It's done for the temporary modification of the body, a stitched reconfiguration of parts that is pleasing to the eye or to the senses. It is versatile, potent and lends itself well to a variety of applications, from algolagnia[1] to artistry.

> The three of them stood in the dungeon, facing one another. If you closed your eyes and looked at them, you'd have sworn they were holding hands. They weren't. The physical symbol binding them together was a simple purple ribbon; the actual connection was much stronger and far less visible.
>
> The other ritual had taken place earlier, at home. Naked they'd sat on the big bed, mingling their blood, using that commingled blood to fill three matching silver vials to be worn as a symbol of their union. They cried a bit, shared laughter and kisses. They spoke their love for each other and their intent to be with each other. They created a connection that

---

1   *Sexual gratification derived from inflicting or experiencing pain.*

time, distance and circumstance could never violate,
no matter what.

In the public space of a dungeon play party, they
stood together, a triangle of support, love and union.
There, in the midst of their community and friends,
in the presence of anyone who chose to notice and
celebrate with them, they affirmed their commit-
ment to each other with one needle apiece, just
above the heart chakra, connected by the purple
ribbon and Everything Else.

PLAY PIERCING ISN'T FOR EVERYONE

If you are diabetic, immune-suppressed, have a blood clotting disorder (i.e., hemophilia), a seizure disorder or vascular
disorder, you'll want to research your condition and the possible
impacts of play piercing before making an informed choice about
participating in this activity. Likewise, if you are taking any drugs,
from aspirin to prescription medication, that thin the blood, slow
coagulation and encourage bleeding you'll want to acquire the
information necessary to make an informed choice. Herbs like
motherwort have the same action. If you're pregnant or nursing,
exercise extreme care and make a deeply informed choice.

If you have a bloodborne illness such as Hepatitis C, Lyme
disease or HIV (to name just a few of the many), make certain to
tell your partner so that they can make an informed choice and
take the appropriate precautions. There are no absolutes when it
comes to who should or shouldn't play pierce, but I invite you to
carefully choose your relationship to this activity.

RISK

There are risks associated with play piercing. If there
weren't, it wouldn't pack such a wallop of taboo. There's physical,

emotional, mental and spiritual risk. One of the most common risks, even among medical professionals, is infection. Local infections are easily treated, but an infection in the bloodstream can run from very serious to life-threatening. Accidental needle sticks make infection just as much of a risk for the piercer as the piercee.

If a needle's not in deep enough or it is used too roughly, it can tear through the skin. Painful bruising (*subcutaneous hematoma*) and swelling can occur if larger blood vessels are punctured. In the worst case, internal bleeding can cause enough tissue pressure in a confined body part, like a finger, to cut off blood supply and cause tissue necrosis (tissue death). Severe consequences are rare, but possible.

If a needle nicks or scratches a bone — highly unlikely, but still possible — it creates an opportunity for bacteria or fungus to reach the bone, or it may directly inserting infectious material into the bone itself. Bone infections are painful, difficult to treat, and may become fatal.

A few cases of MRSA (a dangerous, antibiotic-resistant form of staph infection) have been reported in connection with play piercing. If your immune system is weakened — if, for example, you've had to have an antibiotic shot when having your teeth cleaned — play piercing may not be the sport for you.

Clots and other veinous obstructions caused by invisible bleeding under the skin can cause heart and/or brain trauma, resulting in everything from minor damage that's never noticed to brain damage and death.

Nicking a nerve or disrupting a nerve cluster (a site where nerves intersect and join into larger bundles) causes severe pain and may result in permanent neurological damage; pressure on a nerve from an hematoma can do the same.

Play piercing is a blood sport: any bloodborne pathogen may be transmitted during play piercing, and pathogens like

HIV and hepatitis are of particular concern. If your playmate has something in their blood and you come into contact with it through open skin, mucous membranes, a needle stick or blood consumption[2], the odds are very high that you will acquire whatever your playmate has.

This is not a low-risk activity. Sexually Transmitted Diseases (STDs) are not the only bloodborne pathogen risks; other bloodborne illnesses such as Lyme disease, Ebola and tick-borne Encephalitis are also exposure risks, albeit much, much lesser ones.

There's only so much preparation that can be done to minimize psychological and emotional risk. You may come to understand something intellectually, but until that thing becomes experiential knowledge, it's all in your head. There's no telling what mental doors may be unlocked with a needle; the best you can do is be open to whatever experience presents itself. You may find yourself challenged by "hurting" someone with a needle. You may find yourself completely freaked by being punctured. You may be disturbed by putting a needle in someone. You may remember something long forgotten; you may become aware of something within that you didn't know was there. Those are never bad things; they're the fodder for mental and emotional growth. You can't heal until you learn where — and what — your wounds are. You can't push your own edges until you locate them. When you're an active participant in your own life, you seek those edges in order to expand. When you're not, those edges are terrifying gateways to the abyss. You may experience strong emotions. You may cry. You may find yourself frighten-

---

2   *The primary infection risk consuming blood is not blood in the stomach. Stomach fluids kill most bacteria, and blood is broken down just like any other protein. The infection risk associated with consumption comes from hidden, unknown openings in the mucous membranes of the mouth or upper esophagus.*

ingly "high" from piercing or being pierced. You may shake or shiver. In those moments, breathing slowly and deeply is the best thing you can do.

The spirit should be treated with the same accord offered to mind and skinsuit. It's an inseparable part of the whole and, as such, is subject to risk as well. Spiritual risk lies in lack of intent, in exposing your spirit to unaccustomed rigors without a path of discipline or form of deliberate direction. Spirit is infinitely powerful, and the ego would love to get its hands on some of that power.

Many people use risk — physical, mental and spiritual — to feel powerful and successful. The desire to prove power and success by taking risks doesn't add to one's spiritual growth. What's worse, ego-driven risk taking can lead to a reinforced ego. The ego, however, will not be satisfied with small doses of illusory power and success. The original problem, the need to prove power and success, remains intact. The desire to have more power arises, leading to risk taking as a form of power acquisition instead of a path of surrender to the Divine. Some people climb a mountain and talk about having conquered the mountain; in spiritual terms, the goal is to conquer the self enough to be with and learn from the mountain. If your spiritual aim is to get closer to the All, the Divine, risks that feed the ego through proof of power and success are dangerous.

Another spiritual risk we take with play piercing is the dissolution of the artificial barriers we use to sustain the illusion of separation from one another. If you're not prepared for it, the realization that there is no true difference between you and someone else can manifest as an earthquake in your soul. This phenomenon can rattle you right down to the foundations of your existence and may require serious cleanup. This intensity of connection can make comedown challenging; after spending time in a unitive state, moving back into the "real" world can be brutal and disappointing.

Now that I have your attention, I remind you that all of these risks are commutable with the information you'll find in this book coupled with some common sense: go slow, pay attention, use appropriate precautions and think before you poke. Full disclosure of risk and risk behaviors permits other people to make informed choices in relationship to you; you may not always get exactly what you think you want, but everything you do get will be clean and untainted with the unpleasant flavors of guilt, shame and lies. The power and pleasure you claim will prove worth the peril.

NEGOTIATION

All of our choices should be informed in proportion to the risk. Make sure that you give and get the information you need to make an informed choice about any activity in which you choose to participate. You are responsible for your own health and pleasure. It is your right and your privilege to deliver clear, abundant information and to insist on receiving nothing less.

The best way to make informed choices is to have plenty of accurate information. The best tool to use to get that information from someone else is negotiation. The ability to communicate one's desires, boundaries and limitations is essential to any successful exchange of energy, especially those that involve physical risk.

Keep in mind that it's more difficult to talk about taboo subjects, and play piercing carries a strong taboo with it. Be circumspect in telling your partner(s) what you desire to occur, what you desire to avoid, how far you're willing to go, and where your physical and emotional limitations are. A novice may not know where all their desires and edges are; starting easy and moving slowly will give the novice a chance to enjoy the trial and error of learning without too much error involved. Both piercer and piercee should be honest about their experiences to date and go from there.

Once you know where you're starting from, you can ask questions to help get you where you want to go. Are you allergic to anything, such as topical antibiotics or lubricants, latex or adhesives? Do you want a pain scene or a pleasure scene? Do you want to see how many needles you can take all over your skinsuit, or do you want a certain number of needles in a certain place? Can you take intensity in some places but not in others? Do you have any conditions that can be transmitted by blood? Do you have seizures when things get intense? Do you orgasm from pain? Do you get off on the taste of blood or from having your blood consumed? Can I taste your skin? Your blood?

What will each of you need afterwards? Snuggling and coziness or being left alone to enjoy the comedown solo? Give careful consideration to how you and things you do might impact your partner(s) and share that information liberally. Use negotiations as foreplay; you'll get and give essential information, creating a focus and a bond that will serve you well by helping you make informed choices.

Our preparations near completion. We've looked at the reasons why anyone would want to do this, the risks associated with play piercing on different levels, and how to talk about getting the most of what we want from the experience. We have the internal equipment needed to climb the mountain; let's get started on the journey.

Forty

"Ow!" she said, and jerked just a bit.

"Ow!" she said again, as the next needle went in exactly half an inch from the first six, each neatly half an inch from the other. "Owie owie owie!" she cried,

as the next needle hit a tender spot, and went under her skin anyway.

They laughed. She had a t-shirt that said "'Ouch' Is Not a Safeword" and every time either one of then said "Ow!" or "Ouch!" or their own special "Owieowi-eowie!" it was an in-joke, a private amusement about pain, love and endurance that they shared.

She'd asked for forty needles to commemorate her fortieth natal day. She had never expected to live this long, and each needle was a joyful remembrance of all she had suffered and survived. Ten came and went, with great glee. Twenty came and went, some before the endorphin rush, and some smoothly after. Thirty came and went with a seriousness and calm. They crept towards each other, two lines of twenty needles each, intended to meet over her heart center, right in the middle of her chest. When the time came for number forty, she was ready. She met forty with a smile, happy to still be in the skin that earned her the right to bear her chosen badge of celebration and courage.

FAQ

Does it hurt?

Yes. And no. It's a needle going into your skin. For people who play with intense sensation, this does not register as pain or, if it does, it quickly transmutes itself to pleasure.

Will it scar?

Probably not. The larger the gauge and the longer its in the skin, the higher the likelihood of scarring. Everyone scars differently, and needles only leave small, clean puncture wounds. If there is a scar, it will only be a small dot, unless it was a huge needle, was left in for days, or tweaked on excessively. Learn how the piercee scars by looking at old scratches and the like, then consider the gauge of the needle relative to how they scar. Make an informed choice.

Can I make it scar?

Not so much. Even if you do get it to scar, it's going to be a lot of manipulation and an unreliable result. If you really want a scar, consider something strictly dermal, like cutting for scarification or a larger needle that's used for puncture only, not full subdermal insertion. The more melanin or pigment you have in your skin, the more likely you are not only to scar, but to keloid (large, wide, raised scarring).

Can I pierce through a scar?

Sure, but you shouldn't. Scar tissue isn't the same as regular tissue. It doesn't have nerve cells so it may not have any sensation; what's the point? It can hurt more to pierce it because of its connection to the tissue around it and how that issue is pulled. Piercing a scar can trigger additional scarring or even exuberant scar production which leaves a mass called a keloid formation. You can pierce around a scar, but it's not a great idea to run a needle under it; it's hard to tell from the surface how deep a scar runs.

Can I pierce tattoos?

Yes, if the wearer is willing to risk a scar in their ink. Best to avoid tattoos unless you negotiate the possibility of permanent alterations to them.

Is it okay to pierce freckles?

Yes. Freckles are simply visible concentrations of melanin. It's not okay to pierce moles and skin tags. Moles are non-cancerous collections of cells with pigment; skin tags are the same, but without color. Piercing them can trigger abnormal cellular growth and may prevent them form being accurate indicators of skin cancer.

Can I put a needle under one that's already in the skin?

Yes. But plan ahead if you're going to do that; the first needle should be in deep enough that the second needle won't be pushed out by the distension another needle will cause. It doesn't need to be a whole lot deeper, just a smidge.

Can I do more than one pass with a needle?

Yes, if they're long enough. Plan your entry and exit accordingly if you're going to do multiple passes, or get longer needles. I favor longer needles as opposed to shorter passes because shorter passes are easier to tear.

Can I use acupuncture needles? Or sewing needles?

You can, but you shouldn't. Acupuncture needle are too thin and fine for play piercing. Sewing needles and other sharp shiny objects you may have lying around the house are not clean enough, and may have either coatings that could end up in the bloodstream or faults in the material that can cause a risky subdermal abrasion. Sterile hypodermics aren't expensive or hard to come by; use the right tool for the job. Suture needles are generally safe as well.

Can I use those tiny little pokey things diabetics use?

Sure, if you want to do play poking as well as play piercing. They're called lancets and are small, sharp instruments used to obtain a drop or two of blood. It's unusual for a lancet poke to produce more than a drop or two, so they're not ideal for blood consumption play. They're generally too short to get you into trouble as long as you stay in appropriate play piercing zones, and you can really tenderize the heck out of someone with repeated pokings. They dull quickly, so change them often; they're inexpensive. Dispose of them the same way you would any other sharps.

Can I play pierce in the bath or a hot tub?

Yes, but be advised: the increased temperature of water accelerates the metabolism, as well as decreasing clotting, and you're likely to bleed quite a bit more. The odds of dizziness and fainting are also considerably higher. Sit in water long enough and you get wrinkly; skin in that condition loses much of its oil, which protects against bacteria. The water you're in may be loaded with bacteria, and an open wound is as good as an invitation. If you're sharing water, ask before you get in; not everyone may want to take on the chance of a blood bond with you.

What should I do if I accidentally stick myself with a used needle?

Make it bleed as much as possible to expel pathogens. *Do not* stick your finger in your mouth! While your own saliva is good for your own wounds, you may be putting someone else's juices in your mouth by sucking your own wound. Unglove, wash well with an antibacterial soap and put a band aid on it.

If you push the needle through the piercee and stick yourself on exit, do not immediately pull the needle back through the piercee. You've been exposed to their blood at this point, but they haven't been as exposed to yours.

Here's one method to deal with this situation: Cork the needle and get your metal snips out of your kit. Snip off the hub and pull the needle through in the direction it was already headed.

If the needle is too close to the skin to do this, then flush an antibacterial solution (one part bleached mixed with nine parts water, or Betadine, Wavicide or a similar cleanser) through the needle and clean the available parts of the needle well with the bug-killer.

In any case, go with the piercee to an emergency room or other testing site. The piercee should be tested for disease if they're unsure of their status and you may be treated appropriately for any sticks you've had.

I have asthma and it flares up when I get excited. Can I be play pierced?

Yes, but make sure to tell your piercer that you have asthma and have your inhaler handy. Make sure the piercer knows where your inhaler is as well. You might also want to choose piercers that have a first aid certification.

Do I need a first aid certification to play pierce?

No, but no knowledge is ever wasted and you'll be better prepared to act in an emergency if you have a least basic first aid training. Knowing CPR is never a bad idea.

Can I blow into the end of a needle?

Yes, but the bore of the needle is so small that very little air is likely to get through, even with a larger gauge needle like an 18. Nonetheless, *never* blow into the hub of a needle unless the tip is on the outside of the skin. This is unlikely to cause an embolism — the blood vessels this close to the surface of the skin are too small — but it allows all the bugs in your breath to get under the skin.

Satisfaction — or, The Joy of Getting Your Freak On

The first moment we met, Dan and I had an instant, intense energy exchange. I knew in that moment I had met my evil twin, the person I would be if I had been born male. We live thousands of miles apart, and in the conventional sense, we don't know each other terribly well. As neither one of us are conventional people, I call that a good thing. We see each other once, maybe twice a year. He'd never admit to looking forward to it; he's far too hard and snarky for that. I *suspect he looks forward to it about the same as me; difference is, I don't mind admitting it.*

I managed an extra visit out his way a couple years ago to work a small event he and some good folks had put together. Taught a couple classes, did one of the sickest, wrongest scenes of my life, and got to hang out with Dan and the other organizers after. One of the classes I'd taught was bloodplay, and Dan's a fiendish bloodplayer. Both of us were all hot and bothered by all the fun red sport that had gone on. One of the things I love about Dan is his wit: so sharp, so dry. He starts teasing me about maybe I need to relax, have a few, chill out with the cool kids. I said, "Sure, let's." He reached for his blood kit. I said, "Hey, you said have a few. You know I don't mix liquor and blood; ruins the taste of the blood and harshes my blood high." He says, "Yeah, and I ain't talking beer, neither." At this point, I smell the dare. I picked up the flung gauntlet and said, "Right, as long as you go first."

Since I have a fondness for being on the pointy end of well-wielded needles and appreciate the level of play that comes with years of pleasure in a particular activity, I don't mind getting my fix from a pro. See, he's a needle junkie too. He loves doing it and having it done, just like me. Problem is, it can be tough to find someone with a compatible needle jones. I'm not about to bottom to Dan, and I'm not about to top him. This was more like two friends sharing the love of a fine wine, a sharing of compatible joy.

Keeping with the tone of bravado we'd both set, I said, "All right, asshole, let's go. Put as many in me as you want, but don't put in more than you're willing to take. I receive first. Deal?"

He chortled, truly the evil, maniacal laughter of a sadist about to get his rocks off from both ends at the same time with someone whom he loves to have witty, barbed exchanges.

"Deal. Area?"

"Shoulders, face. No tits." He pretended to pout about that, but he could care less about my tits. That's not the nature of our relationship. I think he pouted because he was certain that heterosexual men are supposed to pout when they can't get their hands on a nice pair or they might lose their Straight Card. He assented.

"You?"

"Same's good. Neck up, and you can just keep your hands of my manboobs too, Missy." Dan makes me laugh. That's why I let him live.

Having chosen weapons and location, it was time to begin the duel. He drew first, as we agreed. My sweet spots are on the top of my shoulder line, from low on my neck out towards my shoulders; his are similar. "You ready?"

"Bring it, Dude. I can take whatever you can dish out."

"Fine," he says, "let's start with some of these nice, pink-hubbed eighteens I have over here."

"Sure, sugar, but just remember: you're next." He chuckled and picked up a twenty-three with a teal hub. "Let's start with these, then. I like the color better anyway, and we can always work up to the pink ones.

Maybe we'll just make you a happy little rainbow of needly pride." We laughed.

He took his visual; I could tell he was plotting his overall design on my shoulders. I know how that look feels on my own face; that showed me how it looked on someone else's. He was a little mean with the first needle; I could tell he was trying to get a rise out of me. I let it work. "Ow, you bastard! Is that the best technique you've got? Maybe I was wrong to permit you to put needles in me!" He semi-sneered, and cocked an amused eyebrow.

"All right, all right, you whinebag. I'll go easier on you. Geez, I didn't realize you were such a puss."

"I'm no puss, you talentless hack, and you know it. You're an inept wannbe if that's all you got. Now show me something good, some style, some flair, before I dismiss you from my presence." That got him good. He started unwrapping the next needle and said, "Well then, I guess I'll just hafta show you how this whole needle thing is really done among true bloodplay-ers." His insert was smooth and in exactly the right place. "Mmmmmmmmmmm," I said as I twitched with pleasure, "Now that's more like it. You may proceed." "When I'm damned good and ready. Now would you please shut up? There's an artist at work, here." "Oh?" I said, looking around the room as he unwrapped the next needle, "I didn't see one. I hope we're not dis-turbing them with all this witty repartee." "Ha ha ha," was his retort as he drove the next needle in. And so it went, for a total of forty some-odd needles in my shoulders.

For added fun, he put a chevron of needles on my chest, five on each side, over my pectorals. That's a great place for needles — and punching. But not both.

Then it was my turn, in much the same spirit of banter, camaraderie and sharp, shiny love, I matched Dan needle for needle. There we stood, facing each other and our respective work, two metallically-plumed peacocks strutting a display for each other. He insisted on taking out the needles in our chests when the display dance turned into a bitch-slapping match; the shoulder needles were out of harm's way, but the chest needles needed to come out. A little light slapping on a piercing is fine, but where we were going was more like pummeling than slapping... so I grudgingly assented to having the pleasurably throbbing needles removed.

We spent the rest of our encounter high on endorphins, surrounded by laughing, cheering friends and beating the crap out of each other.

Section 2: Anatomy

To operate any piece of machinery well and correctly, you need to know something about its parts and how it operates. Play piercing involves the sharp shiny goodness of needles and the stunning intricacies of a skinsuit. Needles are fairly straightforward; skin is a little more complex. We'll look at both.

Anatomy of Needles

Humans come packaged in variety of soft, yummy skinsuits; needles come packaged in a hard plastic shell called a casing. While casings needn't be disposed of in a sharps container[3], you might want to hold on to them until you're done with your piercing session. Uncontaminated casings may be disposed of with regular trash; contaminated casings should go in your sharps or other biohazardous waste container.

Aside from the casing, needles have four parts: the hub, shaft, bezel (some people call this the bevel), and tip. The hub is the plastic cup where the needle would attach to a syringe for medical use and will vary in color by gauge and manufacturer. Hub color can also be an interesting part of multi-needle

---

3   A container used specifically for the containment and disposal of sharp, biohazardous waste such as needles and scalpels.

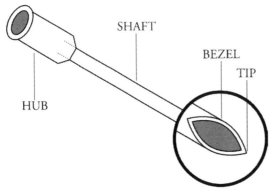

designs and patterns; how might you incorporate color into your design? Pink for a large heart on the back? Blue hubs for the petals of a flower surrounding a breast?

The shaft is the long shiny silver stick that will eventually rest beneath the flesh. The bezel is the slanted edges that surround the opening of the needle, which are incredibly sharp. The tip is the very sharp pointy bit at the end. Despite how sharp they are, disposable needles are manufactured as cheaply as possible and, as a result, dull quickly. If you're going to re-use a needle, limit it to two pokes and only in the same person (unless the pain and tissue abrasion that comes with a dull needle are part of your scene). Never reuse a needle on a different person.

The shaft of a needle is hollow; that makes for a smooth, even insertion, much like a hole punch. The hollow needle through the skin cores a bit of the tissue; this means that the needle itself is not displacing any tissue, so there's less pressure under the skin. Because it's a clean wound and the tissue is removed instead of displaced, unpleasant pain is minimized and optimal healing conditions are established.

To show yourself how this works, try this experiment. Get a piece of paper, a pencil and a hole punch. The pencil is analogous to a sewing-type needle; the hole punch represents a piercing needle. Poke the pencil through a piece of paper, and note the ragged edges and uneven surface that results. If that were skin, you'd have not one wound for the body to heal, but several little jagged wounds, increasing the healing demand on your body and providing more opportunities for infection to get in. Next, pierce the paper with a hole punch and note the smooth, even surface of a single, circular wound. The cleaner the wound, the easier and less traumatic and easier it is for your skinsuit to heal.

The bezel is sharp all the way around, which makes for smooth, even punctures. The sharpness of the bezel also makes it a tool for cutting as well as poking. The bezel is what's being used to score or abrade the tissue beneath the skin. Those edges don't stay sharp for long; use caution when slicing the skin with the bezel or scratching the skin with the tip.

Sizes and Gauges

Needles come in a variety of lengths and gauges (ga). The average length of a play piercing needle is 1.5". For most uses, an inch tends to be too short, and longer needles are often used for more passes per needle and decorative, intricate configurations. Some play piercings, such as stabbings, are done with needles as short as .5".

The gauge of a needle, as with wire or fishing line or anything else that's gauged, refers to diameter or how big around something is. The smaller the gauge of a needle, the higher the number. Twenty seven gauge needles are very fine and thin; for some piercings, they're too flimsy and are far too bendy for pendants or anything hanging from the piercing. Six gauge needles are huge, and almost exclusively used for the insertion of body jewelry. I've never seen a six gauge hypodermic; I expect it would send most people running for the hills. The gauges of generally available hypodermic needles from smallest to largest are: 27, 25, 23, 22, 21, 20, 19, 18, 16, with 16 being quite large for play piercing. Individual preferences will vary, but the average play piercing needles is 1.5 inches long and gauged at 23 or 25.

Some say that the larger the needle, the more intense the sensation. That's true, to a point. Most people can't specifically tell a 27 from a 23, or a 22 from a 20. What people sense is a range. Smaller needles, 27-23, feel about the same. 19-16 ga needles bear a similarity of feeling to each other, but feel a bit more intense than the smaller needles. Experiment; with practice you might be able to teach yourself or your piercee how to tell the difference. The size of the needles does not determine how much pain there will be, but rather what type: in general, thinner needles inflict a sharper, pointier pain while larger needles inflict a deeper, throbbing pain.

ANATOMY OF SKIN

The skinsuit you wear is the largest organ of the human body. It keeps intruders out and your assorted parts in. It acts as insulation, thermostat, radiator and sensory interface. It fully sloughs itself off and regenerates itself every seven years. It's key

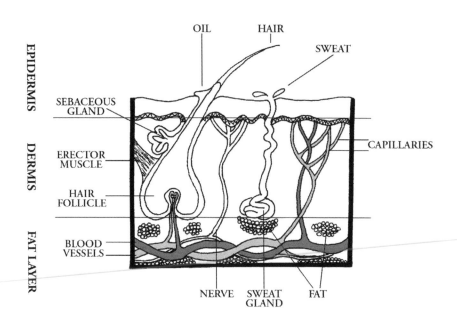

to the survival of your body. For all it does, it's only .07 inches (2mm) thick in most places, although it may vary from .04-.13 inch (1.5-4mm). On average, an adult has from 18-20 square feet (about 2 square meters) of skin, which weighs about 6 pounds (2.7 kg), roughly 4% of your adult weight.

Your skinsuit is made up of three distinct layers: epidermis, dermis and subcutaneous. Play piercings generally go through all three with the majority of the shaft embedded in the subcutaneous tissue, but depth can be adjusted for sensation. Shallow piercings are sharper and higher pitched; deeper piercings have more of a low, resonant thrum to them. On average, the depth of a good piercing is between 1/16 and 1/8 of an inch (16.5-33 mm). The variety of sensation at different depths renders the skin much like an instrument to be played, an instrument with great range under finesse.

The outer layer of your skinsuit is called the epidermis; it's tough, protective and contains melanin, which protects against the sun and gives skin its color. Most of the effort in penetrating the skin with a needle is getting through the epidermis; the two lower layers are not as tough. It's translucent, allowing light to pass partially through it, much like frosted glass. The epidermis doesn't contain any blood vessels but gets its oxygen and nutrients from the deeper layers of the skin. It's waterproof, protecting against the entry of most toxins and bacteria and loss of water from the body. It has nerve endings which signal pain and nerve cells specialized for light touch, which makes it versatile and fun to play with.

At the bottom of the epidermis is a very thin membrane, the basement membrane, which attaches the epidermis firmly, though not rigidly, to the dermis below it. The junction between the epidermis and the dermis is not flat; it undulates like rolling hills, more so in some areas of the body than others. A series of finger-like structures called *rete pegs* project up from the dermis, and similar structures project down from the epidermis. These projections fit together like children's blocks, and help to prevent the epidermis from being easily removed. Networks of tiny blood vessels run through the rete pegs, bringing food, vitamins and oxygen to the epidermis. The dermis contains nerves and nerve endings, both for pain and for pleasure. It has sweat glands, oil glands, and hair follicles or roots and blood vessels.

Under the first two skin layers is fatty tissue, the thickness of which varies from person to person. It contains clumps of *adipose* (fat-filled) cells, larger blood vessels and nerves. This fat lies on the muscles and bones as cushion and insulation, to which the whole skin structure is loosely attached by connective tissues[4], so that the skin can move fairly freely while still protecting your innards.

When it's cold, the skin puckers up in an attempt to conserve heat. Piercing cold-puckered skin hurts more, possibly because of what this contraction does to the underlying connection between dermis and epidermis. Have the room warm enough keep the pincushion's skin relaxed and smooth. During arousal, which play piercing can cause, the blood vessels expand, broadening the sensory capacity of the skin and heightening tactile and subdermal sensations. It feels better and more, and the brain chemicals released during arousal also heighten the experience. Use arousal as a tool; get your pincushion aroused to offset their pain, or leave them unaroused if you want the needles to hurt more. If you want a piercing to only hurt at entry and exit, shoot for getting below the dermis into the subcutaneous tissue. If you want a

---

4   For the sadistically inclined, connective tissue massage is quite painful and of great physical benefit to the recipient. It's a nice skill to learn: helping and hurting all at once.

piercing to hurt more, target the area between the epidermis and dermis, but be advised: that's a very shallow piercing and is much more likely to tear.

Skin also has a "grain" — it wrinkles more easily in one direction than the other. You can see the grain on a piece of skin by pinching it first in one direction, then perpendicular to that direction: one pinch will wrinkle up into a series of lines, the other won't, and the series of lines shows you the grain of the skin. Percings that need to bear weight, such as decorated or anchored piercings, should be placed across the grain of the skin, not with it.

PIERCING SITES

Choose your piercing locations wisely. Places where there's good muscle mass covered by a healthy fat layer are best. Places directly over bone, veins, arteries and significant nerve clusters are the most dangerous and should be avoided. Use your own skinsuit as a guide; think about how it would feel to have a needle placed *there* on *you*. Try piercing yourself first; there's

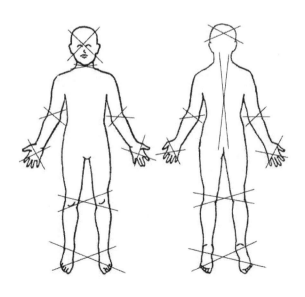

nothing more useful than truly understanding what you're doing to someone else.

Yes	No
Pectoral areas on both men and women	Face, especially the eyes
Breasts	Hands
Shoulders	Feet
Back, but not atop the spine	Neck (base of ears to top of shoulder)
Abdomen	Inside joints (knees, elbows, wrists)
Thighs, all the way around	Over any bone with little padding (shins)
Back of calves	Over arteries
Navel (only innies, never outies)	Depressed areas around the collarbone
Ears (lobes only; avoid cartilage)	From the chin to the front of the neck and down the sternum
Nipples and genitals (need special care; see Section 5)	

John's Dad

Six months ago I decided to no longer tolerate the fifty-five years of conflicted feelings about my father. I resolved to make lasting peace with him. I chose to visit the mountaintop where his ashes were scattered and perform a ceremony of letting go. I chose to carry my emotional pain in the form of a piercing from my home in Wyoming to my destination in California. Removing the piercing on the mountaintop, I would symbolically leave behind all the bad memories, keep the good ones, and thank him for what he gave me. I chose two piercings: one for my pain, and one for my father's. As the needles entered me, I grunted (which was all I could do): "Power and Love, Power and Love."

I felt nearly weightless, saw brilliant lights, and love of the world suffused my heart. I danced, my energy gradually diminished until I sank to the ground to rest. When it was time, I drove to the eastern boundary of Yosemite National Park and hiked to my father's favorite place.

After climbing more than 12,000 feet in elevation I arrived at a high saddle flanked by two rocky headlands. My plan was to camp far above timberline that night, spend the following day in the company of my father, sleep again and then return to the trailhead. I dropped my pack and sleeping bag on the broad gravelly ridge, climbed the higher of the two rocky pillars, and sat for more than two hours soaking in the spectacular view. Mountains, snowfields, meadows and lakes spread 360 degrees around me.

I intended to burn some herbs, a letter of goodbye, some photographs of myself and my family and then combine those ashes with the scattered remains of my father. The wind was blowing strongly; though I struck more than twenty matches I could not light a fire. The wind, which was nearly blowing me off my feet, portended a fierce and probably sleepless night. The angular, fist-sized rocks were large enough to make sleeping very uncomfortable but not large enough to build a shelter. A strategic retreat was in order, but I had unfinished business.

I showed a photograph of myself to the four directions so my father would recognize me. I was ready *to remove the first of the two needles that had been a part of me for the last three days. With the first, I told my father the purpose of this spiritual journey: "This needle represents my pain, my love, and my good wishes for you. I remove it now, leaving all the heartbreak and disappointment which it represents behind me forever." The wind sighed, the trees nodding witnesses. With the second: "I have carried this needle for you, which I now remove, with all its lost promise and pain, leaving it forever." The wind answered with a roar.*

The future will bring new insights, understanding and resolution of my relationship with my father and with myself. I continue to talk to him and thank him for the good things he gave me; we are becoming friends again.

Section 3: Perforation

Technically, all one needs to play pierce are needles and a human pincushion. Technically, a three-year old can use an electric meat knife. Neither is a Good Idea. I fancy myself a risk-taker; you may fancy yourself one also. But infections and disease transmission aren't my kinks. Though there aren't any "rules" to this game, it behooves you to learn how to play thorough and clean; you can always adjust your practice to down and dirty later, if you decide to spin that wheel and take that risk.

The first thing you should always do before engaging in any fluid exchange activity is wash your hands. Put on gloves, clean your surfaces. Change your gloves, set your tray (the preferably portable, flat surface on which you'll place your tools). Change your gloves, prep your pincushion. One more glove change, and you're off and poking. That's the procedure to follow if you want to do this according to medical standards. The common sense angle behind all the glove changes is the prevention of cross-contaminating surfaces, people and objects. Think about what you just touched and what you're about to touch next. If the two things don't go together, change gloves. Even if you're fluid bonded, you may wish to consider gloves. Your fluids may be compatible, but the invisible infection you picked up right before insertion may not be so compatible.

You'll need light to see by. Glaring light bulbs or fluorescent lights don't lend themselves well to a sexy vibe (but they're great for interrogation scenes involving needle threats). An adequate supply of candles will give you sufficient light to work with and may help create that romantic, intimate atmosphere that invites a sensuous experience. The important thing is to be sure you can see well enough to pierce with accuracy. You might want to turn off the phone and put in your favorite music.

Clean your area and set up your tray or whatever clean, flat, preferably portable surface you choose to use. Cleaned well, a baking sheet, cookie tray or the seat of a chair will do in a pinch. For an extra layer of protection, cover your surface with plastic wrap after it's cleaned.

CLEANING SURFACES

The fundamental principle to remember when cleaning surfaces and skin is that any foreign material in the body will cause an inflammatory reaction. If there are bacteria in the foreign material, it will cause an infection. Foreign matter, like soap, lotion and perfume chemicals are likely to cause an inflammatory reaction that can be difficult to distinguish from an infection. The most important way to prevent both inflammation and infection is to clean away foreign material and chemicals first from the surfaces that will come into contact with your supplies and then from the skin that will receive them.

There are a number of supplies available for cleaning the surfaces where you'll be placing your piercee and your supplies. Sterility isn't required for play piercing, but medical-grade products (like Sporicidin) afford you greater pathogen protection than antibacterial wipes you get from the grocery store. Be sure to wipe down your surface after play piercing as well to prevent the transmission of blood-borne pathogens, even if you don't see any blood. Some other recommended surface cleaners are Super

Sani-Cloth, Sani-Cloth Plus and Sani-Cloth HB (the only Environmental Protection Agency approved, pre-moistened disposable wipe that kills the Hepatitis B virus (HBV)). Check online and medical suppliers for more options and choose the one best suited to your practices and preferences.

CLEANING SKIN

The best way to begin is on skin that's clean. Bathing or showering will get you off to a fine start and can also be incorporated into foreplay. After basic hygiene, there are a number of products for cleaning skinsuits; your preference will vary. Whatever you choose, begin at the center of the area you plan to pierce and clean in a circular motion, spiraling outward.

Alcohol (between 70% and 90% isopropyl) is a good place to start. I recommend sealed, sterile alcohol prep pads, not alcohol from a bottle (the risk of cross-contamination is higher). Alcohol used for aftercare will sting. Some people like that, others don't.

Hibiclens or Hibiscrub (clorhexidrine) is a common, broad-spectrum, anitpathogen, pre-operative skin cleaner. So is iodine (Betadine or Povidone), but it's an allergen to some and turns the skin yellow-orange. An allergy to seafood bodes likely for an iodine allergy. Techni-care is gaining popularity; it's broad spectrum, has a low toxicity and low allergen reaction. It doesn't sting, which makes it nice for aftercare but no long-term consequences of its use are available yet. If you're doing this for the blood, use a skin cleanser that won't taste foul or poison you. Choose the product best suited to your needs.

SET YOUR TRAY

It doesn't do to be fishing around in your play piercing kit or toybag for something you need in the middle of a scene. Since it's better to have something and not need it than it is to need something and not have it, even if you don't use them all you'll want to have the following items:

- Surface disinfectant
- Alcohol prep pads or other skin disinfectant
- Fresh, clean gloves made from a material non-allergenic to your playmate(s)
- An assortment of needles in the appropriate length and gauge for your scene
- Surgical marking pen (other ink pens *can* be used, but never gel ink)
- Lubricant (topical antibiotic/anti-infective like Neosporin, Polysporin, bacitracin — generics are fine, but always ask your playmate about allergies)
- Rubber corks, size 000 or 00 or hatpin clutches (both can be sterilized in an autoclave; regular cork will do in a pinch)
- Paper towel, cotton balls and/or gauze squares for prep and clean up
- Peroxide in a squirt bottle for runners and blood clean up (it makes nifty bubbles and gets warm)
- Adhesive bandage strips
- Trash receptacle
- Scissors
- Chux (disposable blue plastic pads) or towels to protect linens, furniture
- Thimble (to prevent sticks)
- Sharps container (a "real" one or a heavy duty plastic bottle with a lid)

(For more details, see Appendix B, "A Basic Play Piercing Kit.")

PROCEDURE

There are two basic categories of piercings: those that go through the skin, either as a surface to surface or as a pinch, and those that go straight in. Straight-in piercings are known as "stabbing" and stabbing is pretty much that: a needle put straight down into the meat, perpendicular to the skin, with no exit point. There are places and conditions under which this technique is acceptable, but that's an advanced technique. Lancets, the very short, sharp shiny things used to provoke small quantities of blood for things like diabetic testing, are an exception and may be used with relative safety for stabbing. Use them on meaty areas only, never over bone, significant nerve clusters or in the face. Lancets are safer for stabbing because they're so short; that also means they're likely to pop out easily as the swelling from the histamine reaction occurs.

The focus of this book is piercings that go through the skin. Whether it's a surface-to-surface or a pinch, there's an entry point and an exit. The procedure for both of those is the same.

INSERTION

Cleanliness during insertion will help minimize the risk of infection. Remember: clean things that touch dirty things are no longer clean. Open boxes and packages ahead of time. Lay things out within reach and think ahead to avoid cross-contamination. Re-glove more often than you think you need to.

There's two ways to insert a needle: smooth and easy or abrupt and hurty. Begin by doing smooth, controlled inserts; expand on that technique once you've mastered it. There are also two ways to brace insertion: with the casing or with your fingers.

Before you poke anything or anyone, the first thing to do is wash your hands and glove up. The right way to wash your hands to reduce bacterium and prevent pathogen transmission is to use an antibacterial soap (naturopathic or allopathic) and water as hot as you can stand it. Vigorously rub and scrub for at least 60 seconds, and don't forget your wrists. Try to make sure that excess water runs towards your elbows, not towards your fingertips so that it carries bacteria away from cleaner areas. Do not touch any surface that has not been thoroughly cleaned between washing and gloving or you'll have contaminated your hands and will need to start over. Dry your hands and forearms well with a clean towel; wet hands are a bitch to get into gloves. Always check with your playmate for latex or other material allergies. Put on your gloves and remain attentive to what you touch.

Next, clean the piercee's skin. Starting at the center of your piercing area, apply your cleanser. While you're cleaning by wiping the skin in an outward spiral motion, look at the skin you're about to puncture. Are there moles, skin tags, scabs, bruises or scars that you'll need to avoid? If you use alcohol, keep in mind that evaporating alcohol chills skin and can cause puckering. Wait for the skin to relax before you pierce. If you're using non-sterile exam gloves, change them after cleaning the piercee's skin.

If you're a novice, I recommend that you use a surgical pen (the special ink won't cause inflammation) to mark your entry and exit, at least at first. It helps to train your eyes to the dimensions that will eventually become automatic. For precision, use a measuring device to mark your half an inch between dots; just make sure the measuring device is clean and in good repair before you put it on clean skin. After a time and with practice, you'll notice that you no longer need the markings.

If you're going to do multiple piercings, remember to work in such a way that previously inserted needles don't interfere with incoming needles. Being right-handed, I tend to work from left to right and top to bottom whenever possible.

The bit of the casing covers most of the hub; the rest of the casing covers the shaft. Pop the hub out of the casing — *just* the hub. Where the hub sits in the casing may be a snug fit; be sure to pull firmly but slowly, or the needle may come out of the casing too quickly and scratch or poke you. When the hub is free of the casing, remove the needle.

Once your small but mighty sword is freed from its sheath, get a good grip on it. The best hold for the hub is the thumb on one side of the hub and your fuck-you finger (the long one in the middle) on the other, using the index finger over the hub for insertion leverage. This hold affords a great deal of stability and control.

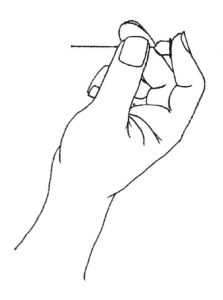

At this point, you may choose to slide the needle through the lubricant of the topical antibiotic you've chosen, covering somewhere approximately one third and one half of the shaft — some experts feel that the lubricant reduces the possibility of infection, while others believe it increases it (since these lubricants are designed for use outside the skin, not inside it). You don't need a huge gob of lube on the needle, just enough to smooth the insertion. If you pierce without the lubricant, be aware that it may hurt a little tiny bit more. If you forego the lube, you won't have to worry about eating antibiotic ointment should you lick around the piercing or indulge in blood consumption after removal.

Whether you mark or simply make note of where you want the entry and exit points to be, position your fingers just to the outside of those spots. Pinch your fingers close enough together to create a firm rise in the skin, but not so hard that you hurt the piercee (unless you want to, of course). Align the needle so that the tip is bezel up, and the shaft is perpendicular to your fingertips. Make sure your horizontal line (the line between the entry and exit points) is where you want it, especially if you're doing patterning. Make sure that your vertical line is parallel to the skin itself. Otherwise, one end of the piercing will be deeper than the other; that sort of leverage increases the chance of tearing.

If you worry about poking yourself with a needle that has someone else's blood on it you can use a metal sewing thimble, cleaned prior to each session, to prevent a stick. You may also use a cork or the needle casing at the exit point. To do this, put the cork or the mouth of the casing directly over the exit point. It can be tricky to hold something at the exit and still support the entry point; you may wish to practice this technique on a chicken breast or a plum before you poke a person.

You've set your marks, or made note of freckles or lines on the skin to use as landmarks. You've checked your alignment and your bezel is up. You're ready to push the needle through the skin. Now is a really good time to check in with the piercee. Make eye contact, and ask them to breathe with you. I recommend three good, deep breaths that originate low in the belly, in through the nose and out through the mouth; not only does breathing connect you to your pincushion, it relaxes and prepares both of you for the experience. Deep breathing may also increase the oxygen in the bloodstream, enhancing sensation and aiding in pain processing,

It usually takes at least one breath for them to synch up with you. If their breathing is fast, erratic or very high up in the chest, they are anxious and may not be ready for the pierce. Make more eye contact, and offer reassurance in words, touch, or both. Try again with the three deep breaths. Meditative breathing as an adjunct to play piercing also ups the odds of making the piercing experience more deliberately transcendent. When your breathing is synchronized, return your attention to the piercing site. Take another breath and pierce on the exhale; piercing on the exhale is generally easier on the piercee.

We were full of silly seriousness that expressed itself through giggling and smiles. We were little kids playing a secret game. We breathed together. We were lost in our own world. I felt her move through me with each breath we took; at first, inhaling and exhaling together. Then she switched it on me: she inhaled as I exhaled, drawing in my old breath to become her new one, offering me her breath to sustain my next inhale. It felt tidal, as if we took turns being the ocean and the beach. Waves of her washed over me, and I held her breath for her.

She took the needle to my skin as she watched and felt my breath. She pushed the needle through my skin and as it entered me, I felt it was she who had penetrated and entered me. Every time she pierced me with a needle, she entered me. As I felt the pain come into me, she felt the pain she inflicted on me and we moved with an energetic flow like water. We shared love, heat, intensity and arousal. As I got high off the endorphin rush from the piercing, she got high from my high. As she got high, her sadistic and child-like glee intensified and I felt love flowing through her to me and back again. The intensity of our connection, heightened by the breath, took us over the edges of our selves and into the forever place.

While you're exhaling together, push the needle through by applying even pressure while keeping the needle parallel to the skin. Push firmly and gently. Go slowly, smoothly, evenly, watching the needle move beneath the skin as it heads towards the exit point. The needle is sliding through the fatty layer during this stage of the piercing and there's very little pain. The first piercings generally hurt more than subsequent ones; it can take a few to get the endorphins rushing well.

Piercing the exit is usually more painful than the entry because the skin is more stretched. Before you break skin at the exit, make sure the needle's point is where you want it to be. You'll be able to tell if you're on your mark by the way the needle distends the tissue. Get your fingers out of the way and make the exit. If you're using a cork or the casing to brace your exit, push the needle through the exit point and into the cork or casing. Settle the needle under the skin so that you see a sequence of shaft, skin, shaft in mostly equal parts. Cork the needle or use a hatpin clutch if you're in public or need to for any other reason.Repeat as desired. After some practice, you'll be able to perform an insertion rapidly while still taking all the factors into consideration.

How Deep?

The needle should rest approximately 1/8th to 1/16th of an inch (3.3mm to 1.6mm) beneath the skin. Any deeper and you're messing with muscle meat. Shallower than that and the entire path of the needle will cause pain. At a shallow depth, the skin is more likely to tear if it's accidentally tugged. It's not an easy exact measurement to take; the best gauge is a combination of looking at the needle and the skin it's under, listen to your pincushion and feel the resistance as the needle slides through.

There should be a slight but firm, visible mound of skin over the needle. If there's no mound, no contour of flesh to show that there's a foreign object beneath the skin, you're too deep. If you can see the needle through the skin, it's too shallow. To check by feel, run your fingers over the embedded needle. You should feel the rigid hardness of the needle evenly surrounded by softer human tissue. If the piercee claims much pain, it may be too shallow. When the needle slides through, you should feel the resistance of skin, less resistance as it slides through fat and then the resistance of exit. Practice will broaden your piercing vocabulary.

How Long a Pass?

If the needle is the recommended 1.5" (38 mm) long, the embedded section should be roughly one third the full length of the needle. If the needle is too short, you can't pierce enough skin to keep it in place. When skin is pierced, it reddens and swells. This is a normal and healthy response to invaders. The swelling that results from normal inflammatory responses can, however, swallow a needle that's too short, leaving the point beneath the skin. That can cause abrasion you may not desire and cannot observe. Whatever your choice of needle length, there should be enough room on either side of the embedded metal to prevent the needle from being forced out by inflammatory swelling. Usually, a half-inch (~13 mm) pass is sufficient. The appropriate length for a pass is determined by the overall length of the needle; the pass should be one-third of the overall needle length.

Subdermal Sensation Techniques

Once the needles are in the skin, you have some options. You can play nice, and just let them sit. You can play mostly nice, and just touch the skin gently as it rests over the shaft. It's a fascinating sensation, that small rod of metal under the skin. Unless a needle is moved or otherwise impacted, the primary sensation will be the initial rush of insertion followed by a deepening warmth and tingle as the rush fades.

Not everyone wants to play nice. There are some things you can do that are not so nice, like thwacking a finger on the skin above the shaft. Repeatedly, if you like. You can hold the hub in one hand and the cork in the other and lift the needle gently. The thinner the gauge of the needle, the more gentle you should be; thin metal bends easily, and a curved shaft affects how the needle is removed. Extreme pullings and tuggings are redundant and potentially harmful. Gentle movements are really all you need to seem very mean indeed, because the sensation is already intense. Keep an eye on endorphin responses; stacking pain on top of pain will deepen the rush but it may also cause a bigger post-scene crash for the piercee.

Subdermal abrasion (using the tip of the needle to abrade the tissue under the skin) can be quite painful. Don't do it accidentally, and if you do choose to do it, be prepared for additional soreness and bruising as well as a longer healing time. The risk of infection is also higher; you're reinserting part of the needle that's been exposed to contaminants and you're scoring tissue you can't see. If you lift up on the hub of the needle, you're using the tip to score the dermis closer to the fat layer. There are more blood vessels here, and the bruising that results will be deeper and last longer. In fact, you may not even see an immediate result from the scoring, other than more blood on removal. If you want additional scoring, twist the needle so that the bezel is facing down.

If you push down on the hub, you're using the bezel and tip to score the dermis and epidermis. This produces a higher, sharper type of pain and is quite irritating as well as likely to result in more immediate visible bruising.

DECORATING

Ribbons, laces, bows, dangly bits: the limit is your imagination—and the tensile strength of your pincushion's skin. If you choose to augment your work in any way, make certain that all of your art supplies are cleaned and disinfected. Choose your cleaners according to whether or not the ornaments will be going into the skin or on it. If you're going to string fishing line through a piercing, don't clean it with a surface disinfectant.

If you leave the needles in the skin, you can wrap ribbons or string around them to create anything from a mandala (we called them "god's eyes" at summer church camp, and we made them with popsicle sticks and yarn) to a "corset" (lacing around piercings much as one would lace, well, a corset). You can string beads on a cord between two needles. You can use long needles, take more than one pass per needle, and weave feathers into the metal gridwork. You can bind two piercees together, and have them pull on each other (a fine ritual/ecstatic technique). If you're going to hang things from needles, use a larger gauge needle (22 ga and larger) so that the metal beneath the skin does not bow when dependent weight is added. For more elaborate designs, think it through ahead of time. The direction of the needles, their placement in relationship to each other and the extra materials for your design are all factors to be considered in advance.

Leaving the needles in also allows you to insert things into the hub of the needle, using it as a miniature vase. I've seen everything from flowers (dried, artificial and real) to small bunny ears used for hub stuffers; choose the items that are right for you. Sacred ritual items might be small crystals or feathers; playful intimacies might warrant beads with faces painted on them or perhaps antennae. Feel free to get creative, but make sure everything is clean before it goes near the piercing.

Another option for décor involves fishing line and removing the needles. This technique requires that you make sure your needle is big enough in gauge to accommodate the line; I recommend a 23 or larger for this combined with the right gauge of fishing line. Soak the line for up to 12 hours in a cold sterilant like Wavicide 01, then wash it carefully with distilled water. After inserting the needles, insert the fishing line through the tip of the needle. Pull it through the hub, and then remove the needle while holding the line. Be advised: though it can (and *should!*) be cleaned, fishing line cannot be completely sterilized. Use at your own risk. If you leave the ends of the fishing line long enough, you can tie bells, balls, baubles or whatever you like to the line. As a rule of thumb, especially for beginners, do not exceed one pound of weight per piercing and watch the piercing very carefully to make sure the fishing line doesn't pull through the skin. Pulling through skin may leave a scar, and the tear should be treated as a wound. If you're wondering whether or not the wound needs sutures, go to the emergency room.

If you're fascinated by string under the skin with things hanging from it, I encourage you to explore learning to suture. Though no better or worse than fishing line dangles, suturing is a simpler technique than threading fishing line through the small end of a needle, and sterile sutures can be obtained at any medical supply house.

Though not exactly decorating, predicament bondage can be done with needles, and it's certainly beautiful. Run needles up the fore and upper arms, along the outside. Do the same with the outer thighs and calves. Lay the pincushion face up. Using longer strands of ribbon, six to ten feet, lace the pincushion like a shoe starting at the top of the upper arm all the way down to the lower calf. It's gorgeous, and the pincushion isn't about to go anywhere the piercer doesn't want them to. For additional effect, roll the pincushion over and repeat the lacing from the back.

Kat's boy didn't much care for needles. He had a hard time processing that particular type of intensity. To his credit, he was willing to overcome and try to eroticize his own pain so that he might be of greater pleasure to Kat. He wanted her to be happy all over him, whether he liked it or not.

Kat didn't much care that her boy had a hard time with needles. She had a vision of his stocky, muscular back pierced, punctured and perforated with a grid of metal lines to be woven with the object of her choice: feathers.

Kat wanted to fly by giving her boy wings. We chose 3" 18 gauge spinal needles; at that length, each needle could make two passes, creating a more stable foundation for the design as well as having the aesthetic advantage of fewer hubs showing. We chose a diamond criss-cross pattern over each shoulder blade with about an inch and a half clearance on either side of the spine. The grid layout perfectly matched the contours of his shoulder blades and back lines. Kat wanted the wings to seem as if they'd sprouted fully formed from his own skin.

He was stoic. He climbed up on the massage table, settling himself in for a nice, long ride. When he stopped fidgeting, we took our positions, me on the left and Kat on the right. We each placed a hand on our respective shoulder blade and breathed with him to start the circuit of energy running. We reached for needles, set our marks. He breathed in, and we pierced him on exhale, again and again and again. He struggled, we laughed and sighed. He endured eighty four double pass insertions, which added up to one hundred sixty eight holes in his skinsuit. He grunted and groaned like someone moving heavy things, using sounds to tell us that he was rearranging his consciousness to make room inside of himself for all the intense sensations. Play party and watchers fell away; it was just the three of us, some music and the pile of waiting needles we'd laid in the small of his back.

We worked on him in timeless space for what the clock said was an hour and a half. Kat had chosen white feathers for his wings; black would have looked misplaced on his tanned, blond, construction-worker skinsuit. We used two bags of smaller feathers towards the top of the wings and a bag of larger ones at the bottom to resemble pinfeathers. He lay altered on the massage table, looking like he'd been pounced on by a feather monster. The weaving turned out beautifully; very little metal could be seen through the feathers. There was nothing to disrupt the illusion.

The last feather found its home. Kat and I stood back arm in arm, admiring our handiwork. Kat bent to his ear, asked him something. "Yes, Ma'am, " he muttered. "He's ready," Kat told me in her cool, confident voice, and "Ohmigawd, I'm about to have a fantasy come true," she told me with her gleeful, sequined eyes.

He rose. Slowly. He eventually stood, exploring his rearrangement with each small movement that makes up a bigger movement. He moved with care, noticing how his new features affected his old, deep ways of moving. His breathing came and went in short huffs, holding against the pain, releasing when there was none, holding on to his tension as support for whatever pain might be lurking in his changes of position, releasing the tension on exhale. He stood firm, exhaled a mix of relief and satisfaction with his pain and turned his gaze to Kat. He was beatific, alight from within, some foreign, new glow illumining the golden hue of his skin.

I told him to shrug. He looked at Kat; she nodded, smiling. He closed his eyes, concentrating, trying to feel for a shortcut around how much he expected the movement to hurt. Realizing there was no way around the pain, only through it, he moved. He lifted and lowered his shoulders. A smile bloomed on his face as he realized that the pain he expected was indeed there, but bearable, even loveable. His soul took flight in that moment as he realized that not even his own pain, inflicted by another, was enough to stop him from fulfilling a commitment. He became the angel he resembled; his wings lifted him on a new pulse of beat and rise, beat and rise. Kat and I soared with him, riding the current of overcoming and transformation on brand new wings.

54

Section 4: Tidying Up

Removal

When?

Needles can safely be left in the skin for approximately twenty minutes. That's an average; your mileage will vary. Any foreign object that disrupts the integrity of your skinsuit will eventually trigger an inflammatory response. Normally harmless body chemicals congregate at the site of the intrusion and attempt to repel the invader. The immune system, the body's self-defense mechanism, reacts to foreign objects and substances that invade it. Inflammation brings more blood and lymph fluid to the site of invasion, which act to bring more immune cells there to help fight the "intruder" and more blood flow to help carry away poisons. In some people, but not all, the immune system is hyperactive, and over-reacts to certain foreign things. This is called an allergy when it's mild, or "anaphylactic shock" when it is so severe that it can kill you, as in extreme reactions to things like bee stings. The piercee's inflammatory response should be the guide for how long to leave in a needle. You can slow down the response by cleaning the skin well and using an anti-infective lube, like Neosporin, polysporin or bacitracin. Be sure to ask about allergies to topical anti-infectives before using them.

A mild response produces a light shade of pink around the entry and exit. As more of the chemicals congregate at the piercing site, the pinkness will spread to include the section of skin above the needle as well. The area then will continue to redden as more blood and other skinsuit soldiers are called to the site of intrusion. Eventually, the swelling and pressure will increase to the point that the tissue immediately around the entry and exit points will start to pale and whiten. When that happens, it's time to pull the needles out. Be aware that the longer a needle is left in, the greater the risk of infection becomes; the longer the skin is left open, the higher the risk of an uninvited guest finding its way in.

How?

Always brace the entry (the place where the needle went in first) when you remove a needle. It's a tight fit, that needle under the skin, made tighter by the pressure of inflammation, and pulling on the needle drags tissue. You're not going to turn the skin inside out or anything crazy like that, but the pressure of skin being pulled like that can be quite unpleasant. Hold the hub, and use your thumb or forefinger to apply gentle pressure beneath the needle. With practice, you'll learn how much pressure to apply to keep the skin balanced between the extraction and the bracing.

If you feel nice, grab the hub, make sure your trajectory is a straight line, and pull quickly but firmly. To prolong the magic of a gentle removal, pull slowly and evenly.

If you feel mean, grab the hub, tip it, and pull really fast. Tipping the hub scores the tissue along the path of removal, causing more pain and better bleeding. Because a hard, jerky or tipped removal with scoring adds to the pain, it may trigger one last endorphin rush (if there are any endorphins left to be released). If you want more blood, push the needle in and out a few times while tipping the hub up; there are more blood vessels towards that fat than there are towards the epidermis. If the histamine response is already strong when you go to remove, no matter how rough you are you're going to get less blood because of the swelling. If you want a good bleeder, remove sooner and then tip and score.

Once the needle is out of the skin, immediately dispose of it in a sharps container or heavy-duty plastic bottle with a lid. Sharps containers can be purchased in a variety of sizes at drug and medical supply stores, or ordered online. In lieu of a sharps container, use a heavy-duty plastic bottle with a lid (something like what fabric softener and detergent come in) and put used needles in it. When it's full, duct tape the lid shut and clearly mark it with "sharps" and "biohazard." You can then take it to your local waste management plant or landfill for disposal. In some places, pharmacies will accept full sharps containers for disposal and even exchange the old for a new.

CLEAN UP AFTER YOURSELF

The cleanup process is where most wound contamination takes place, and with you and your pincushion both flying high, it's time to be extra-careful.

You may get blood in places you didn't expect to, and you may get no blood at all in places you thought you would. Odds are, you're going to get some blood somewhere. Letting blood run over sensitive skin is a rush. If you're a hemophile, play with it, but keep in mind that blood dries much faster than Hollywood would have you believe. If you're going to play with it, do so quickly. If you're going to consume it, do so even more quickly. Congealed blood at room temperature loses a great deal of its comestible charm.

If you get a bleeder you don't want, or one that's reluctant to stop, use a sterile gauze pad to apply pressure to the wound. Hold the pressure until the bleeding stops, which it will; the wounds caused by play piercing simply aren't that large, unless you've done something inappropriate. If the bleeding doesn't stop after pressing for a while, you may not be pressing the right spot or you haven't pressed long enough. Cover the entire area of the pass and press firmly for five minutes as the clock flies. This will stop almost any bleeding.

If the blood is spurting, you've hit an artery. Arterial bleeding is stopped the same way as veinous bleeding, but it takes longer (about twenty minutes) and is riskier. Arteries carry blood to the parts of the body that are even further from the heart than the injuries you've caused. Pressing hard enough to stop arterial bleeding means that the artery isn't carrying blood downstream. If you cannot stop spurting blood within a minute and a half, go to an emergency room immediately.

If you've followed the guidelines for where and how to pierce, you're unlikely to hit a major blood vessel. If you've decided to perform riskier piercings and have sought hands-on education to that end, you're unlikely to make the mistakes that come with the arrogance of assuming something that looks easy is simple. If you've done it appropriately, you should have a non-infected wound and just enough blood to play with, eat, or fingerpaint with. After all, for many of us, a little bit of blood is part of play piercing's charm.

As much fun as playing in blood can be, dried blood can be challenging to remove. Some piercers prefer sterile saline wipes for cleaning up after play, but my favorite method of cleaning blood off skin is a squirt bottle of hydrogen peroxide. It oxygenates the blood, making it bubble as it pleasantly heats the skin. Once loosened by the peroxide, the blood lifts right off (it's also good for getting fresh blood out of fabric, followed by a cold water rinse — however, it'll bleach hair and remove color from dyed hair).

AFTERCARE

Give your pincushion water to drink. Water may be the single most important facet of aftercare, closely followed by warmth and snuggling (if that's what works for the piercee. Ask). Some protein and something sweet are always good after heavy endorphin play of any sort. Cheese, meat, crackers, fruit, chocolate: all fine items. Of course, you negotiated ahead of time what your piercee might need in the way of aftercare, so you know if it's snuggling or being left alone, protein or fructose that works. Take good care of your toys and they'll be more likely to play with you again.

Not all aftercare is physical. If you exercise your skinsuit, you get sore in places unaccustomed to such activity. The same rule applies to moving your energy and your psyche around. Perhaps you've done a scene with only three needles. Not such a big deal for the skinsuit, right? But what if those three needles were symbolic of three intense losses or pains, and they were positioned over the second, third and fourth chakras? If you've used a play piercing experience as a vision quest or a means to catharsis, remember that the parts of you less visible than your skinsuit will require aftercare as well; you may be tender in those places for a while, especially if those parts of you are unaccustomed to rigorous activity.

Whatever the specific form of aftercare is, be sure to honor the journey and what you've shared. It's important to note that it isn't always just the piercee who has an endorphin crash; that can happen to the piercer as well. Remain present and attentive; you can't go wrong with compassion and communication.

The spent needles blinked arhythmically in the gut-
tering candlelight. The sheets were disheveled; the
cuffs lay unbuckled and opened, flaccid at the ends
of the chains. Their breathing sounded more like one
person in stereo than two people breathing together.
They were unified, sewn together by the invisible
lines in, around, between each of the needles he'd
just removed from her flesh. It was their anniversary
and he'd wanted to gift her with something special.
He had been afraid to give her needles, even though
he knew she loved them, even though he'd seen her
wide smile and glazed eyes when she talked about
them. He'd faced his fear not for her, but because
of her. He discovered with the first needle that on
the other side of his fear lay a gorgeous innerscape
of connection and engagement. He'd always enjoyed
hurting her, but had never known it could be like
this. She'd hoped he could take her to that place
with him, she'd dreamt it was possible, and now she
knew.

They inhaled deeply, exhaled with a sigh, and then
laughed together at their identical timing. He opened
his eyes to see her staring up at him. He kissed her on
the forehead, and handed her the water. She smiled;
he'd read her mind. She drank, and set the glass on
the night table. He smiled, knowing that she needed
little aftercare if the scene had been intense. She
knew that when he pushed her envelope, took her to
a place that stripped her of her illusions and left her
clean, he was usually exhausted. She needed a little
water, some chocolate in about twenty minutes. He

needed to make sure she was all right, and then he'd cry a little and have some ice cream. It was his release. She wanted him to know how she honored what he'd given her—not just the needles, but the overcoming of his own fear. She knew he'd used her as a catalyst to overcome his fear; in a way, the piercings had been his way of thanking her for helping him to learn more about himself. He was thankful that she had the grace to let it look like it was all his idea. They held each other just as closely in the space after as the space during; without judgment or comment each gave the other what was needed, in love and in joy. He made room inside himself for her desire and its pointy ambassadors. She accepted his gift, and they both got bigger.

TROUBLESHOOTING

Most of the troubleshooting to be done with play piercing is psychological and emotional. Done correctly, it's difficult to cause severe physical harm by play piercing alone. On removal, you might get a bleeder; as with any other wound, apply pressure until the bleeding subsides and stops. It also helps to elevate the wound site above heart level.

Should you require medical attention, do not allow your fears to become shame. Tell the medical professionals exactly what you were doing and how the injury occurred. Doing so enables them to treat you most effectively and preserves your own integrity. Show them, by example, that there is nothing wrong or shameful in what you do in the privacy of your own life.

Medical attention is required if:

- You get a bleeder that won't stop.
- A bruise turns into a knot beneath the skin and continues to swell for more than a couple of hours and doesn't respond to ice or anti-inflammatories.
- A hole you thought was closed become hot, red and/or inflamed and is accompanied by swelling, an odd yellow or greenish discharge, a funny smell or a fever.
- You notice a line of redness leading away from the piercing site; it's an indication of blood poisoning.
- You experience continued, prolonged neurological (nerve) pain emanating from or connected to a piercing site.
- A needle or fishing line rips through the skin and stitches are required. A wound may be irrigated and bandaged with SteriStrips at home *if* it is no deeper than the dermis, not over a joint, is not contaminated and is no more than ½" - ¾" in length. Watch closely and carefully for signs of infection. If in doubt, seek medical attention.

Allergic reactions can run from a minor skin irritation to hives to severe anaphylactic (no breathing) shock, which is far more likely to be a reaction to a cleanser or lubricant than it is to the needle itself. It's rare to have a first-time extreme reaction; most people know if they have an allergy and presence of allergies should have been thoroughly addressed during negotiations. Seek immediate medical attention if the piercee suddenly exhibits fast, pronounced swelling, hives, itching and/or difficulty breathing.

Some people faint. If you get a piercee or voyeur who does, do not keep them in a sitting or standing position; that can be dangerous. Lay them flat with the head at or below the level of the heart and elevate the legs above the level of the heart. Check their pulse and breathing; if the pulse drops below 40 beats per minute, call 911 and watch them constantly. People recover rapidly from fainting if placed in the right position. When they recover, don't let them get up immediately; keep them down and quiet for 15 to 20 minutes; offer water when they feel able to drink. Help them to first sit, then rise if they're alright. When they're ready to stand, stay near in case of dizziness or another faint.

Seek emergency medical help if:

- They don't come to within five minutes.
- They hit their head or something else on the way down.
- They complain of chest pains, persistent pounding heartbeat, can't see correctly, can't speak or can't move limbs.
- They convulse, seize or lose bowel control.

Basic Wound Care

The three basic principles of wound care are:

Keep the wound clean.

Keep the wound moist[5].

Keep the wound well nourished with blood and oxygen by reducing or eliminating swelling and keeping pressure off the wound.

If it happens that a needle tears through, clean and dress the wound. Wash your hands and change gloves. Gently flush the wound with water to clear out any foreign matter and bacteria. If inclined, you can do a peroxide rinse as well, remembering to rinse the peroxide with water when you're done. Apply a topical antibiotic ointment (you have some in your kit, right?) and use the appropriate bandage to cover the trauma site or to pull the edges of the skin together in the case of a tear. Cover that with a larger gauze and tape bandage. If the wound requires stitches, head for the emergency room. If it doesn't, keep the wound clean and change the dressing once a day for three to five days. When

---

5 Keeping a wound moist or dry is climate dependent. In most arid and temperate places, it's best to keep a wound moist. In extra-humid places, it's best to dry the wound as quickly as possible.

the wound is closed and a healthy shade of pink, it no longer needs bandaging.

He hated needles. Absofuckinglutely hated the goddamned things. It wasn't a bad experience at the phlebotomist's. It wasn't a childhood trauma involving sharp things. He just flat out didn't like the way the steely little bastards winked at him when they came out of the casing, as if they knew they were going to taste a piece of him and there was nothing he could do about it.

When she pulled out her blood kit, that safety-orange Black and Decker toolbox purchased to accommodate her bloodletting supplies and covered with Happy Bunny stickers, he always shuddered. If she stopped at the first tier of the box for a lancet, a quick and simple nip, all was well. Those went in quick, a pinprick, and she could usually make that small puncture bleed just enough to keep her happy for a while. If she removed the first tier and dug a scalpel from the second tier, he heaved a sigh of relief. He didn't mind scalpels; the pain was clean and he scarred beautifully. He was proud of how well he held her marks. She never put a mark on him that she wasn't willing to look at for a lifetime, and that built trust. But when the second tier came out on the heels of the first, he cringed. There was only one thing at the bottom of that box, underneath the instruments he'd made peace with: needles.

He hated the needles, but he took them for her. He took them for the satisfaction of feeding her, of being her Food. He took them for the expressions of ecstatic bliss and maniacal glee that crossed her face when she slid the little buggers under his armor.

Mostly, he took them because he loved her, and she loved needles. Somehow, that made it all okay. He could find a way to cope with the intense sensations. He could find a way to deal with his dislike of the menacing barbs. What he couldn't do was find it within himself to deny her something of such great joy, just because he didn't like it very much.

66

Section 5: Advanced Practices

Play Piercing and Blood Play

"Everywhere one looks, there flicker the shadows of primordial struggles: the perpetual tension between the dark and the light; the wrestling match between Christ and Satan; and finally, the complex allegories of sex: sex in all its unimaginable innocence, or sex reeking with the full perfume of the swamp. And all these urgencies are seen or sensed through a hot wash of blood which, deny it though we will, fascinates us very nearly to the point of shame." — Leonard Wolf

Play piercing generates wonderful consequences. There's the aesthetics of a pretty needle design on skin, the endorphin rush (for the piercer as well as the piercee), and, of course, blood -- red, wet, slick, sticky, warm, tasty blood. Where there's blood, fetishists and vampires will appear.

A fetishist is aroused by a particular object or circumstance; some folks have a shoe fetish, some have a fetish for flashing. A vampire, for the purpose of this discussion, is one who consumes blood (fancy black clothing and morbid angst optional). The balancing and necessary companion to vampire is donor, one who is emotionally and physically gratified by providing blood for the vampire. Donors are not victims; that's a different type of roleplay. A donor is empowered by the knowledge that what they contain is sacred and desired. The healthy exchange between a donor and a vampire recognizes that the two do not, cannot, exist independently of each other, that both are required if either is to be fulfilled.

Not all vampires are blood fetishists; some vampires prefer only to sup and are not sexually aroused by blood consumption. Not all blood fetishists are vampires; some fetishists enjoy a tactile or visual experience with blood while never desiring to taste it.

I am a vampiric blood fetishist. I am eroticized to blood and many of the methods of its extraction. I am emotionally and sexually aroused by blood; the word for someone like that is *sanguiphile* (*sanguis* is Latin for blood). Someone who sups on blood is a *sanguivore*. Blood fetishism is my cake and I like it with vampire-flavored icing.

Coincidentally, I am a sadist; I enjoy inflicting pain for the removal of blood from its living, breathing carafe. Blood is a fine and heady wine that breathes always.

I am not confused about the difference between my imagination and my reality (though I do enjoy deliberately blurring those lines from time to time). I am not a member of the undead masses, I do not expect to live forever, shifting from one identity to the next, lifetime after lifetime. I don't expect to live longer than my current forever, during which time I shall age ever so gracefully and decline into mature sophistication. I fantasize that I shall be old, recumbent upon a divan in the conservatory and have flutes of fresh blood brought to me be dedicated, nubile younglings.

I appreciate and have much considered the symbolism of the vampire archetype[6]. To entertain a vampire is to invite the Shadow in, to entertain a manifestation of death, the ultimate transition from the known to the unknown. There's risk, fear and the concurrent excitement of doing things we're not "supposed" to. When we play with the energy of a vampire archetype, we're playing with a transition from the known to the unknown, and to make that transition deliberately is taboo.

The power embedded in a taboo is naturally strong; it must be in order to act as a self-regulating method of social control. Some taboos, like not urinating in public, are a good idea: hygienic treatment of bodily wastes inhibits spread of disease, keeping everyone safer and healthier. Other taboos, like those around sexuality, at one time may have served a general social purpose but many have outlived that purpose. When we break a taboo, whether in private or public, we take the lid off that enormous can of power and have at our disposal a tremendous creative force with which to sculpt a public scene, a private interaction or anything else we desire.

Vampires are an archetype that reflects the use of enormous creative power without guilt or shame. A victim is selected, exploited, and abandoned. That association between omniscience and impunity is attractive. No harm can come to a vampire in myth, film or imagination. In play, the rush of power exchange, the donor's vulnerability, their permission to be violated simulates the illusion of being impervious to harm and fosters the intimate connection of joining with another being in sacred communion.

Archetype: An original model or type after which other similar things are patterned; a prototype; an ideal example of a type; quintessence. In Jungian psychology, an inherited pattern of thought or symbolic imagery derived from the past collective experience and present in the individual unconscious. Fodder for myth.

Life feeds on itself: things live, grow and die, becoming something else or food for the next cycle of growth. Acknowledged or not, we are a part of that cycle and crave its manifestation in our lives; the vampiric paradigm through the power of the myths associated with it and the universal truths in the archetype.

It is not "safe" to play with power as strong as the stuff that imbues the vampire archetype. Many people have issues around blood and bloodletting that squick them; blood as a symbol represents an essence of life that carries within it phenomenal power. So much power, in fact, that blood is a part of every known recorded religion. Religions are attempts to make sense of the world and a tool we use to establish a sense of order in the chaos. Blood flows through all of those attempts contained between the banks of the sacred and profane.

It all comes down to power. It may begin with crafting an environment of soft lights and sweet music to help set the scene for a vampiric exchange. We sometimes need external reinforcement in order to be able to enact our dreams, visions, cravings, fantasies. Soon, though, the strength of the archetype begins to fill the exchange and it becomes its own thing. There is no room for anything other than the people involved and the blood between them. In BDSM, that power and its exchange is honest and clean instead of sneaky and dirty; we admit we want to play with power and seek ways in which to do so that don't get us retaliated against or arrested. It's a paradox: we seek ways to safely do the unsafe. We seek the edges of ourselves without getting too close to the edges drawn around us by history and culture.

We can create safer ways to play with power, but there is no safety net with blood. If blood is ingested, transmission of any bloodborne pathogen is all but 100% guaranteed. If not ingested, blood can be handled with caution and safety to minimize transmission risk, but there is no known way to eliminate risk in bloodplay. Vampirism is a dance of passion on the razor's edge of risk, and one's dance partner may be Death. That particular edge, that rush is part of what makes bloodplay so very, very potent.

Blood is potent. Play piercing is, too. If you play pierce for blood, use larger needles and irritate the tissue. Don't leave the needles in long enough for the histamine reaction to turn the area around the piercings white; that's an indication of low blood flow to the area and you won't get much juice that way. The best time to pull needles is when the site is red and inflamed. That's an indication of increased blood flow to the area.

The places many people associate with bloodletting are terrible for play piercing. *Please do not ever for any reason stick needles in anyone's wrists, inner elbows or neck near the carotid arteries or jugular veins.* Certain areas of the body tend to produce better than others; upper arms and thighs are good. Meat and fat in abundance and balance are what you're after for good production. Production is affected by body temperature; cold people don't bleed as well because the body is conserving heat by pulling blood towards the core and organs, away from the skin. Alcohol and aspirin encourage bleeding by thinning the blood, but they leave an aftertaste and should be used with caution to prevent inappropriate blood loss.

Multiple sticks with lancets on meaty areas like the chest over the pectoral muscles can be productive, but then you have tiny droplets over a wide area instead of one or two good centralized bleeders. The distribution of wounds and blood is a matter of personal preference. I suggest avoiding menstrual blood as food; it's dead blood, being used by the body to slough off dead tissue and doesn't taste good. It's great for art projects, though.

As with standard food, it's not just what you eat, it's how much. Small amounts of ingested blood (a teaspoon or less) are unlikely to produce any unpleasant results. Many consumers find that eating more than a teaspoon or so can cause nausea and vomiting; blood has an incredibly complex protein structure and can be challenging for the stomach to break down in large quantities. For each quantity of blood a vampire ingests, the donor has lost that much blood. One can safely lose about a pint, and that much loss will probably make a donor woozy and a vampire sick from "overeating." Any greater loss than a pint and bone marrow can't generate enough new blood to replace what's been lost. It's unlikely that high volumes of blood will be shed from play piercing.

Everyone's taste varies — literally. We truly are what we eat, and the flavor of blood reflects one's diet, physical activity levels and degree of hydration. Blood tells many stories. People who don't drink enough water taste silty and metallic. Part of the job of blood is to remove toxins in the system to waste disposal sites; without enough water to aid in that task more debris stays in the blood and makes for an unpleasant taste. It's recommended that one consume roughly half of one's overall blood volume in water per day, about two and half liters. Copper and iron both have very distinct flavors in the blood and are far more pronounced in a dehydrated donor. Many supplementary vitamins and minerals will also leave a taste.

Most blood-drinkers report that vegetarians taste different than carnivores. Their blood generally tastes cleaner, but it's not as rich. Vegetarian blood is more like blood light. Vegan blood is terribly bland but very clean. Carnivore blood is rich and more flavorful, but varies depending on other components of the donor's diet. Donors who eat a lot of fatty and fried foods taste greasy. Too much fast food makes a donor taste like, well, fast food. Not enough vegetables and fruit in a carnivore's diet makes them taste like yesterday's hamburger. Folks with high cholesterol levels taste like gravy. People who eat fish more than twice a week taste fishy.

Everything one ingests flavors the blood: food, beverages, medications all leave behind a tasteable trace. If medications are involved, discover how long and in what form they remain in the bloodstream. The timeframe of ingestion plays a part also; it takes about an hour after ingestion for the flavor of food to affect the blood. I favor having a donor eat some meat (usually beef), a nice mixed-greens salad (not iceberg lettuce) and some chocolate, with maybe a little red wine. Chocolate-and-port blood is delicious, but watch how much sugar is being ingested. Oversugared blood isn't all that pleasant and too much sugar makes the donor more likely to faint. Have your donor eat or avoid certain foods; play around with your favorite flavor combinations. Please your vampire by concocting a recipe to flavor your blood in interesting, tasty ways. A healthy, well-balanced diet not only makes you taste better; it makes you feel better about yourself and the world around you. Adequate rest and sufficient exercise also contribute to yummy, flavorful blood.

Physical aftercare for vampire or blood fetish scenes is similar to the aftercare for any other type of scene. Water, rest, some fruit juice, some protein; all will help to stabilize and ground the skinsuit and its contents. Emotional aftercare for any intense scene is going to involve heightened communication. I invite you to negotiate the specific type of aftercare that works for you, and to communicate your needs and desires clearly.

> She said, "I'm hungry." I knew what She meant. When She'd expressed Her hunger before, it was time for me to leave. She fed only from Her donor and never in front of me. She would play with me, arousing Herself on my body while her donor watched; then She'd send me away, hungry and hungry.
>
> I rose to leave. She stopped me and told me to fetch The Box. I had never been allowed to touch the

dark, carved wooden box that held Her bloodletting supplies but I knew exactly where it was.

She took needles from the box and laid them on the table. She summoned me to the cushion at Her feet. The twin to my cushion was occupied by Her donor, his head in Her lap, absentmindedly stroked, light scratches of manicured claws raking to and fro across his shoulders. She cupped my chin, turning my attention towards Her. As I turned, I caught Her donor's eye. He smiled, both blessing and assent.

She opened Her box, removing a knife. I shuddered. I held myself in check; no matter how She chose to feed, I would not dishonor this privilege by dictating the experience or running away from it. She would have me any way She liked.

She held the knife to my throat, above my pulse. It jumped from my neck as though it were straining to reach the edge of the blade. She drew the point downward and my world narrowed to the point of that blade. She preferred to unwrap Her food with a knife. She waited, Her unspoken request to cut my clothes off hovering between us like a firefly, a question made of light and possibility. No bra and tee shirt was worth the price of losing this moment.

With peaceful excitement and anticipation, She cut my clothes from me, the only trace a pile of white cotton shreds on the floor.

She reached for a needle with Her hands and for me with Her eyes. Had I wanted to move, I could not. She smiled again, and warmth suffused my skin and soul. She would accept me tonight; She would take me in Her embrace and make me part of Her. I would be with Her always, singing my own note in the music of her life. I was ready to take that responsibility.

She pierced me over my heart, on the left side of my chest. The first needle was a sharp sweet sting of indrawn breath. The second was a heated cousin of the first; the third, a vibrant sigh of edges. The fourth was a hot knife through cool butter; the fifth a burst of every yes I'd ever said. She surveyed Her work, touching me everywhere with her approval. My skin hummed, my cunt ached. No penetration I'd ever felt was quite like this; my cunt was hungry and fed at the same time.

She touched the needles, moving them, twisting them so that I'd gasp, patting them gently so that I'd sigh and close my eyes. My eyes closed and She opened me, removing all five needles quickly and brutally. I arched, screaming. She pulled me into Her lap, my body arced over Her thigh and I felt Her hair touch my skin a moment before Her lips came to me. She sucked on Her wound; it was my flesh, from what I could remember about what it felt like to wear skin, but the wounds and the blood it held were undeniably Hers. I had only been holding them.

I felt Her moan touch my skin as gently as Her hair had. She sucked harder; a second moan reverberated through me with a rush of heat and passion. I felt something touch my side; it was Her donor's head, his buzzcut fuzzy prickly soft against me. He was going down on Her, feeding her cunt with his mouth and tongue. That pleasure made Her wounds two-way *streets; my blood coming out and her sex going in. The energy rose, built, spiraled upwards. We rose together, the world falling away from all of us together more than what any one of us was alone. We collided in the air, each of us riddled by the shards of union and dissolution. We fell back to the here and now where we began, breathless, bloody and at peace.*

NIPPLES AND GENITALS

Play piercing is intense. Genitals have lots of intense pleasure potential. Combining the two intensities is an alchemy that's both heady and dangerous. I'm aware that even high-risk piercings have been performed for a very long time and in conditions far less hygienic than our modern civilizations. I'm not trying to reinvent the wheel; I'm trying to prevent people from being run over by it. Please, if you choose to pursue nipple or genital piercings, do so with the utmost forethought and caution.

If you're a new, novice or amateur piercer and you opened this book up to this section thinking to start with the juicy bits right off, I invite you to slow down, back up and go read the other stuff first. You'll need the specific piercing techniques elsewhere in this book in order to do a successful genital piercing. If you're an experienced play piercer, incorporate this information thoroughly into your existing skillset and techniques before you proceed.

Statistically, the odds may be in your favor that you could pierce a nipple or a labia or a cock and have nothing go wrong, but you should give some serious thought as to whether or not you're truly willing to take the risk of having someone's nipple lose sensitivity, get someone's cock infected and become impotent or have part of someone's labia fall off because it became necrotic and died. You are just as susceptible to worst-case scenarios as anyone else, and your own ignorance is a piercing's worst enemy. Go read the other stuff and come back here later. Think before you poke.

Genital and nipple piercings are some of the most talked-about piercings; they're the sensational ones because they most obviously connect piercing and sex or sexuality. They're also some of the more dangerous piercings. They are not, however, the most intense or gratifying piercings by default. I vehemently advise you against attempting these piercings without additional education, instruction and supervision. These higher-risk piercings each have their own special guidelines but are performed with adaptations of the techniques we've already discussed. Nipple and especially genital tissue has much higher vascular action than other tissue and is more likely to bleed profusely both during and after play piercing.

NIPPLES

Nipples are surrounded by a circular area, usually darker in color than the person's skin, called an areola. It varies per person in size. The little bumps on the areola are Montgomery glands; they produce oil that lubricates the nipple/areola complex. Behind the areola are milk glands and milk ducts as well as fatty tissue. There's no muscle in a breast, other than a few small erector muscles in the nipple. The milk glands feed into the milk ducts, which go all the way into the nipple, opening out to the surface of the skin.

Male and female breast structure is the same. In women, the milk glands develop and become productive; in men, they do not. Gynecomastia is the phenomenon of enlarged breasts on men (manboobs) and is fairly common. Contrary to popular belief, male nipples are just as likely to be sensitive to erotic stimulation as female nipples. Likewise, piercing them is just as risky.

Piercing a nipple disrupts the milk ducts. It can puncture, perforate and sever the ducts. Needles are relatively small and milk ducts are many; occasional play piercing is acceptable and unlikely to cause severe, long-term damage. If you're female and plan to or are breastfeeding, keep play piercings in the nipple to an absolute minimum, perhaps even declining to have your nipples pierced until you're through nursing.

Nipple piercings can cause minor to total loss of nipple sensitivity. If you have sensitive nipples, be aware that piercing them may cost you that sensitivity. If you rely on nipple stimulation to achieve heightened arousal or orgasm, that loss could be painfully significant. Yes, play piercing nipples is a hot idea and a nice rush, but think about whether or not it's worth losing any sensitivity you already have. If your nipples aren't overly sensitive piercing them can actually serve to wake them up, increasing the sensitivity, but that's less likely to occur than loss of sensitivity. Infections can occur, but that's true with any play piercing. Loss of sensitivity is bad, but the worst-case scenario with a wrong nipple piercing is that blood flow to the nipple is disrupted and the nipple becomes necrotic and dies.

If you're going to pierce a nipple, do exactly that. Pierce the nipple, not the areola. The needle should go through the

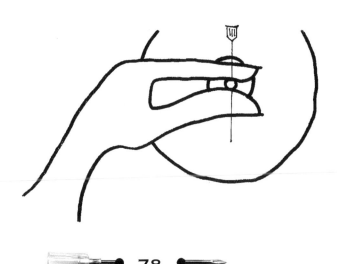

base of the nipple, parallel to the skin of the areola. The closer you get to the tip of the nipple, the more it will hurt and the higher the risk of the needle ripping out. Ripped nipples are excruciatingly painful, are a high risk for infection, and never heal back to quite the way they were. The piercing technique for a nipple is the same as other parts: brace your exit, align your marks both vertically and horizontally, and insert. Ensure that the needle is seated in the middle of the nipple.

MALE GENITALS

The risks associated with male genital piercings are relative to the two large components of pierceable male genitalia: the cock and the scrotum. The balls themselves should *never* be pierced for any reason whatsoever. *Never* stick a needle directly into a testicle; there's no such thing as a "minor" testicular infection and more dramatic consequences, such as a ruptured testicle, are possible. All of the problems that can result from piercing a testicle are nasty and undesirable. Wrong cock piercings can result in infection, tissue collapse, impotence or necrosis; I've never met anyone with a cock who thought that those conditions were a good idea and sounded like fun.

Circumcised cocks have two basic segments: the shaft and the head. In the case of an uncircumcised cock, you also have the foreskin to play with. The head of a cock has a lip or ridge to it, called the corona. That ridge is pierceable, but painful. If you pierce the corona do so from the bottom up, from the underside of the corona towards the tip of the cock, keeping the needle parallel to the shaft. A needle too close to the edge of the corona could result in a rip or tear. Go slowly and proceed with great caution.

The shaft is also pierceable, but only for surface-to-surface piercings. *Never* stick a needle straight through a cock; vascular tissue and the urethra (the tube urine goes through) can be damaged causing severe, painful and expensive health care issues. Cock piercings should be done with plenty of light. Examine the shaft of a cock and you'll notice an intricate web of blood vessels just beneath the skin. Shaft skin is much thinner than skin found elsewhere on the body; it rips easily. It takes a good deal of practice and expertise to calculate how to make a piercing deep enough to prevent ripping and shallow enough to preserve the underlying tissue. At the same time you're calculating depth, you must also be acutely aware of the blood vessels that need to be avoided. Do not pierce blood vessels in the shaft of a cock.

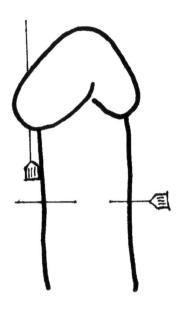

The scrotum warrants the same caution as the shaft; it, too, is riddled with blood vessels that should never be pierced. Surface-to-surface piercings may be done on the scrotum as well as piercings that grab a piece of it and go through, just as with an earlobe. To make sure you're missing all the blood vessels, hold a flashlight up to the scrotum from behind; the scrotum becomes translucent the light will show you where it's safer to pierce.

FEMALE GENITALS

The play pierceable parts of the vulva are the inner labia (or lip), outer labia and clit hood. *Never* put a needle point in the vagina or pierce anywhere near the vaginal opening. The infections that can result could lead to severe complications, including pelvic inflammatory disease, which can in turn lead to severe vaginal and uterine complications including infertility and, in the most extreme cases, death.

Never stick a needle in a clit. *Ever.* The potential risk of sensitivity loss is terribly high. I do not advocate clitoral play piercings nor do I recommend permanent clitoral piercings. If you have a clit you'd like pierced, please seek out a piercer with tremendous amounts of maturity, wisdom and experience. Handle all female genital tissue gingerly. It has a great deal of tensile strength; it's meant to stretch. But the skin itself is rather thin and easily abraded.

The clit hood can be pierced, but only with extraordinary caution. You're dealing with delicate tissue and a very small space in which to put a needle and the clit hood is right next to the clit itself. At its apex, the hood connects to the clit itself. The base of the hood blends into the labia. Piercing the hood creates the risk of nicking the shaft of the clit. Elevate the hood as much as you can from the clit itself by gently pinching the skin down around the shaft of the clit, making sure you can feel the shaft between your fingers. When you feel the shaft slip out of your pinch, you'll know you have only hood in your hand. Use something like a piercer's receiving tube or a clean stick like a tongue depressor inserted between the clit shaft and the hood to protect the clit from being grazed by the tip of the needle. Use a bit of lubricant to make sure nothing sticks to, pulls or abrades the shaft, but don't use too much or your protection will slide out.

Labial configurations vary wildly. Some women have little to no outer labia; some have little to no inner labia. Both inner and outer labia are pierceable in some interesting and intense configurations.

Piercing the outer labia is usually surface-to-surface but, depending on how plush the labia are, it may be done by gently pinching a section of the labia and piercing the tissue as one

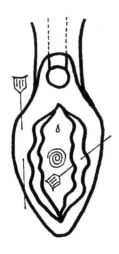

would an earlobe. There's a lot of fat in the outer labia as it's part of the padding protection system for the underlying bones; that fat provides cushion for needles. Mind where you point the needles and the angle of insertion. Needles pointed outward can prick the thighs. Needles pointed in can prick the other labia and perhaps the vaginal opening. Corking the needles in labial piercings is a very good idea. If you find corks too cumbersome, use hatpin clutches.

Piercing the inner labia requires more care. Surface-to-surface piercings should not be done on the inner labia; they're too thin to support that technique and using it is likely to rip a lip. There's even more blood flow in the inner labia than the outer; using the flashlight technique will help you see where the blood vessels are so that you may safely go through the labia. Pierce the inner labia closer to where they attach to the body; the closer you get to the edge of a lip, the higher the risk of a tear. Torn inner labia, like nipples, never quite heal back to their original state. Labia with scar tissue is less sensitive and more prone to additional tearing later on because the tissue on either side of the scar is weakened.

> ... *Rip, pop, poke. "Nineteen." Rip, pop, poke. "Twenty." Rip, pop, poke. "Twenty-one." Rip, pop, poke. "Twenty..." push, grunt, "... two."*
>
> *Needles make noises. The paper they come packaged in rips. There's a "pop" when they exit the casing. There's a "poke" noise made when the needle comes in contact with a person; not like a sealed Tupperware or somesuch, more like a grunt of acknowledgement.*

Needles make people make noises, but there's one particular noise that only emerges when the pincushion has taken the last needle they're going to take. He made that sound somewhere in between "twenty" and "two."

Twenty-two needles isn't all that many. It's a respectable quantity, though hardly excessive. Twenty-two instances of having a needle go in; twenty-two instances of having a needle come out. Endorphins usually kick in around the fifth needle; it can take hundreds of needles to truly tax the endorphin system. Twenty-two is just beginning to think about getting serious. Unless, of course, those twenty-two needles are in your cock.

One of the nice things about cocks is that they get bigger and harder with the appropriate coaxing (the same thing can be said of clits, but it's inadvisable to put twenty-two needles in one of those; it's inadvisable to put any needles in one of those without extreme caution, care and expert knowledge). Pleasure helps to offset the initial shock of a needle; in fact, heightened pleasure can go a long way towards transforming pain into pleasure. But after a nice bout of fellatio, a needle isn't — can't be — anything other than something of a shock. If you're the one with the cock, the shock is hard. If you're the one with the needle, the shock is delicious — so blissful that you shudder with it.

Twenty-two needles make a cock look a little crowded, like a porcupine trying to hide by crawling up into some poor guy's abdominal cavity.

The spongiosum cavernosa is the name of the tissue that creates a stiff cock. Blood engorges the tissue and a hard on is born. If something is done to reduce arousal, the blood vacates the tissue, and the cock gets soft. Some of the blood stays, though, and when those needles come out, the blood comes with it, turning an ordinary, everyday cock into a vampire's dream sucker.

* * *

We all start somewhere, and the end of this book is an invitation to your beginning.

Where will you go from here? Will you hone the ability to hurt people with ever-increasing creativity and grace? Will you explore how to create pain and turn it into pleasure so deep and wide that piercer and piercee alike get lost in a sea of sensation? Will you weave pretty pictures with skin and metal? Will you decorate a living, breathing Christmas tree? Will you hold space for a release of grief and sorrow? Will you rejoice in celebration? Will you give someone their wings and help them learn to fly?

Wherever your journey leads you, I wish you perilous pleasure, pain, power and happy poking!

Appendix A:
Universal Precautions

Universal precautions are infection control guidelines designed to protect people from exposure to diseases spread by blood and certain body fluids. Most of it is common sense; I include it here for your use and reference.

Universal precautions should be followed when exposed to blood and certain other body fluids, including: *Blood, semen, vaginal secretions, breast milk, synovial fluid* (joints), *cerebrospinal fluid, pleural fluid* (around the lungs), *peritoneal fluid* (abdominal, gastrointestinal), *pericardial fluid* (heart), *amniotic fluid* (fetal cushioning). Universal precautions should be applied to all body fluids when it is difficult to identify the specific body fluid or when body fluids are visibly contaminated with blood.

Universal precautions do *not* apply to: Feces, nasal secretions, sputum, sweat, tears, urine, vomitus and saliva (unless it has blood in it).

1. Barrier protection should be used at all times to prevent skin and mucous membrane contamination with blood, body fluids containing visible blood, or other body fluids (cerebrospinal, synovial, pleural, peritoneal, pericardial, and amniotic fluids, semen, breast milk and vaginal secretions). Barrier protection should be used with *all* tissues. The type of barrier protection used should be appropriate for the type of procedures being performed and the type of exposure anticipated. Examples of barrier protection include disposable lab coats, gloves, and eye and face protection.

2. Gloves are to be worn when there is potential for hand or skin contact with blood, other potentially infectious material, or items and surfaces contaminated with these materials.

3. Wear **face protection** (face shield) during procedures that are likely to generate droplets of blood or body fluid to prevent exposure to mucous membranes of the mouth, nose and eyes.

4. Wear **protective body clothing** (disposable laboratory coats (Tyvek) or surgical operating room gowns) when there is a potential for splashing of blood or body fluids.

5. Wash hands or other skin surfaces thoroughly and immediately if contaminated with blood, body fluids containing visible blood, or other body fluids to which universal precautions apply.

6. Wash hands immediately after gloves are removed.

7. Avoid accidental injuries that can be caused by needles, scalpel blades, laboratory instruments, etc. when performing procedures, cleaning instruments, handling sharp instruments, and disposing of used needles, pipettes, etc.

8. Used needles, disposable syringes, scalpel blades, pipettes, and other **sharp items are to be places in puncture resistant containers** marked with a biohazard symbol for disposal.

Simply put: if you're not fluid-bonded, wear gloves (ask about material allergies before you play). Don't get body juice in your eyes, mouth, nose, genital mucosa or open skin. Wash your hands before you don and after you remove your gloves. Don't stick yourself and put used sharps in a safe place. Do yourself one more favor: get tested regularly for all bloodborne illnesses and STD's if you're going to. These tests can often be performed at low to no cost by Planned Parenthood or your local health department.

Appendix B: Resources

There isn't a lot of information about play piercing out there, and most of what is out there is either incomplete, inaccurate or both. That's why I wrote this book. Still, no knowledge is wasted and it can't hurt to read up and make up your own mind.

Cleo DuBois' "The Pain Game" affords an intense, intimate look at play piercing; I highly recommend it.

www.sm-arts.com/paingame.htm

www.sexuality.org/l/bdsm/needle.html

en.wikipedia.org/wiki/Play_piercing

www.bodyplay.com/

www.sandm.com/index.php?p=169,215

public.diversity.org.uk/deviant/ssplyprc.htm

www.safepiercing.org/piercerLocator.php

www.ringsofdesire.com

The Center for Disease Control has useful information about bloodborne pathogens:

www.cdc.gov

See also the World Health Organization:

www.who.int/en

Fakir Intensives is a California State Registered Career Training Instituion for those who wish to learn basic and advanced body piercing techniques, shamanic body piercing, piercing physiology/anatomy and professional health and safety procedures.

Fakir Intensives
PO Box 2575
Menlo Park, CA 94026
Phone 650-234-0543 FAX 650-326-BODY
www.fakir.org

If you're interested in exploring more of the spiritual adaptations of play piercing, try these:

Radical Ecstasy, Janet Hardy and Dossie Easton. Greenery Press, San Francisco, CA, 2004.

Anatomy of the Spirit: The Seven Stages of Power and Healing, Carolyn Myss, Ph.D. Three Rivers Press, New York, NY, 1997.

Why God Won't Go Away: Brain Science and the Biology of Belief. Andrew Newberg, M.D., Eugene D'Aquili, M.D., Ph.D., Vince Rause. Ballantine, New York, NY, 2001.

The Art of Ritual: A Guide to Creating and Performing Your Own Rituals for Growth and Change. Renee Beck and Sydney Metrick. Celestial Arts, Berkeley, CA, 1990.

SUPPLIES

Kinky Medical
www.kinkymedical.net
877-537-1495

Kinky Medical serves the BDSM/Fetish community with a wide variety of medical supplies including needles, scalpels, saline inflation, catheters, instruments, sounds, disinfectants and much more. Their service is fast and friendly.

Rainbow Rope

www.RainbowRope.com

516-608-4550

A wide array of supplies and very friendly; if they don't have what you want, they'll look for it.

BMEZine Shop

www.bmeshop.com

Body Modification EZine was one of the first and remains one of the largest, most comprehensive sources for body modification information.

Play Piercing Kits

www.playpiercingkits.com/

The Play Piercing 101 booklet they offer is adequate though limited. They offer kits; if you want everything all in one package without shopping around, it's a good deal.

92

Appendix C:
A Complete Play Piercing Kit

For easy reference, here's a list of everything you might possibly need during a play piercing scene and a suggestion for where to get the items. Tool and tackle boxes make great containers and are easy to find and relatively cheap. For specific online supply sites, please see the resources section.

What	Where
Surface disinfectant	Online, drugstores, medical supply
Alcohol prep pads or other skin disinfectant	Online, drugstores, medical supply
Fresh, clean gloves made from a material non-allergenic to your playmate(s)	Online, drugstores, medical supply
An assortment of needles in the appropriate length and gauge for your scene	Online, medical supply, some farm and veterinary suppliers
Surgical marking pen (other ink pens *can* be used, but never gel ink)	Online, medical supply
Lubricant (topical antibiotic/anti-infective like Neosporin, Polysporin, bacitracin – generics are fine, but always ask your playmate about allergies)	Drugstores
Rubber corks, size 000 or 00 or hatpin clutches (both can be sterilized; regular cork will do in a pinch)	Hardware stores, online
Sterile gauze squares for prep and clean up	Grocery and drug stores
Hydrogen Peroxide and a squirt bottle for runners and blood clean up (peroxide makes nifty bubbles and gets warm when it contacts blood)	Grocery and drug stores

Adhesive bandage strips or gauze and tape; SteriStrips and Butterfly closures	Grocery and drug stores
Trash receptacle	Anywhere; a recycled grocery bag will do
Scissors	Anywhere
Metal snips in case a needle needs to be cut	Hardware store
Chux (disposable blue plastic pads) or towels to protect linens, furniture	Online, medical supply, drug stores
Thimble, to prevent sticks	Sewing and crafts supply
An assortment of decorative items: ribbon, fishing line, dangly bits, feathers	Sewing and crafts supply, hardware stores, anywhere your imagination goes
Sharps container (a "real" one or a heavy duty plastic bottle with a lid)	Online, medical supply
Lancets	Drug stores, online

96

Acknowledgments

This book is dedicated to those luscious freaks who've pushed the envelopes before me and those who will continue to ask, "How do I do that?"

I offer hearty gratitude and thanks to:

My Mother, who in all likelihood will never read past the title page. She always told me I could do anything.

My Mate, Lawerence. I'm all in, Darlin'. Thanks for continuing to say yes.

My girl, Amy. For her diligence in editing and gentle, consistent persuasion, I award a whole bunch of doughnuts. I have been enriched by your service.

Michael and Alesia; thanks to you, here's another one. The big one's coming.

Kris, amanuensis and friend. Thanks for everything, you lovely whore.

My ed, just because of who you are and the man I see you becoming. I love you.

Grin and Slick, incomparable loves and lovers. I am bigger because of you.

Dr. Chuck Clanton, for medical consultation and enthusiastic commentary. I am blessed by your generosity and playful spirit.

Arielle. With the thanks also comes the Spider Award: here's to conquering fears. Thanks for stepping so willingly into my web.

Rumpledforeskin, for a beautiful tale.

Misty, because she already knows and reminds me gloriously, flamingly.

Silas and Jana, for drinking deep with me. Love to you, oh my brothers!

Ellin Beltz, for the deft editing and keen writer's eye.

About the Author

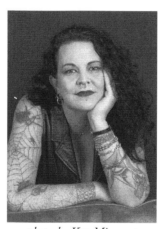

photo by Ken Mierzwa

Deborah Addington is a professional pervert. She teaches a variety of alternative sexuality classes and writes books to assist others in the expansion of their sexual and spiritual horizons. She's a body modification artist, scarification being her speciality, and an ordained minister in the tradition of Modern Mysticism. On the outside, she's a hard femme, six feet tall, dark haired, green eyed, tattooed and pierced. On the inside, she is hungry for knowledge of all sorts, irreverent and extremely frolicsome. She's deliciously sadistic, dominant in service and enjoys living on her own edge while encouraging others to find theirs.

She lives in California's rural and exquisite far Pacific Northwest where she keeps her sanity intact by working with local sex-positive organizations, writing and walking on the beach. This is her third book.

For more information or to make an inquiry about scheduling a class or modification:
Deborah@FistAndFangs.com
www.FistAndFangs.com

Deborah Addington
PO Box 99
Trinidad, CA 95570-0099